The End of Acne

How Water is the Cause of the Modern Acne Epidemic, and the Cure

Melissa Gardner

$\frac{P}{F}$

The information provided in this book is designed to help you make informed decisions about your health. It is intended to be used for informational purposes only, not as a medical treatment. Please consult a knowledgable healthcare provider if you suspect you have a medical problem that requires medical treatment.

To my mother

"...behind all your stories is always your mother's story,
because hers is where yours begin."
—Mitch Albom

"I'm speechless. It all makes sense now. Your face is my face. I can't believe I've never heard of this before."

—*Lauren* from Plano, TX

"I really can't thank you enough for writing your book. Now I know how to protect myself and put a halt to this pain."

—*Alex* from Chicago, IL

"It totally made sense. I cried."

—*Amber* from Bethlehem, PA

"I feel like I have been hitting my head against a brick wall. Thank you so much for writing about this."

—*Stacey* from Canton, IL

"Thank you for this labor of love and info. It's what I have been praying for for a very long time. (Yes, I actually pray about my acne…)"

—*Marie* from Port St. Lucie, FL

"Yup you've got this figured out. GENIUS!"

—*Perry* from Chicago, IL

"Stumbling across your website was a light bulb moment. It is the most likely explanation I have encountered in thirteen years of searching for answers."

—*Erin* from Little Rock, AK

"Your book saved my life. A million times thank you because you helped me avoid going crazy."

—*Irene* from Houston, TX

TABLE OF CONTENTS

Don't forget about this part —it's important!

A Note to the Reader

"YOUR BOOK SAVED MY LIFE." These were the words I received in an email from a woman who read a free guide I posted online in 2011 about how I cured my acne. That weekend I started writing this book so the truth about acne could reach a wider audience.

When I began submitting *The End of Acne* for publication, these are the words I received in an email from a literary agent: "This clearly is a story that needs to be told. My concern is that most publishers would probably want you to be a PhD." I was also told it would take a year or more for these pages to reach the shelves. I know what it's like living with acne, so I didn't think you would want to wait that long. Instead of waiting on the publishing industry, I decided to submit this book to you directly.

As a self-published author, I tried my best to create a book you would enjoy reading but you might still spot some errors in my grammar and formatting, etc. (I admit I mixed up style guides in the footnotes and then left it that way intentionally as an act of defiance. I'm tired of following someone else's random rules of perfection.) If you catch an error that you feel needs to be corrected, please tell me about it by emailing Edit@ProjectFree.Me instead of writing about it in an Amazon review. But please do write an Amazon review, especially if this book helps you with your acne!

Also, if you want to help get the word out about how to heal acne, I am happy to pass on to you a portion of the proceeds from each sale of this book you help generate. Find out more at **ProjectFree.Me/spread-the-word**.

Oh, and you might want to look at the footnotes.[1] Thanks for reading *The End of Acne!* :)

---

[1] I tried to put a lot of good stuff in here, like raisin jokes and direct links to source material so you can draw your own conclusions about the information discussed in these pages. You can also view the footnotes and other references in a .pdf (with active links to journal articles) at **ProjectFree.Me/References**.

INTRODUCTION

The Story of Acne

WE TELL OURSELVES SCIENCE IS KING, but our understanding of the world is shaped through story. We tell stories about the past and call it history. We tell stories about the present and call it news. Our stories about how to act, think, and live are called culture. And our stories about how the natural world works are called science.

We can tell science is a story because of how it changes over time. The earth is flat. Now it's round. Airplanes are impossible.[1] Now they are commonplace. The natural world didn't change, but our understanding of it did. It would be naive to think our current story is a complete picture of how things are.

The story of acne commonly told today goes something like this: when your pores become clogged with dead skin cells and other debris, they trap oil and bacteria in your skin causing an infection in the form of a breakout. The story has variations. Sometimes hormones are involved, sometimes they are not. Sometimes genetics are involved, sometimes they are not. Sometimes diet is a trigger, but everyone is different. One aspect shared by these common stories of acne is the ending—there is no cure for chronic acne, only ongoing treatment.

Every story has a story*teller*. Like a musician conjuring a new piece of music into existence, it is the storyteller who decides who the main characters will be, where the story will start, how it will end, and every detail in between. The storyteller is responsible for deciding which storylines to pursue, which to disregard, and which will be overlooked entirely. In most cases, a story has multiple storytellers

---

[1] Lord Kelvin, an esteemed mathematical physicist regarded for his work formulating the first and second laws of thermodynamics, declared in 1895, "Heavier than air flying machines are impossible," eight years before the Wright Flyer took flight.

whose voices weave together in a cacophony of overlapping assertions and ideas. It is up to the audience to decide which version to retell.

With the story of acne, the dominant storytellers are dermatologists. As physicians who specialize in disorders of the skin, dermatologists pull their main characters from their textbooks: pores, skin cells, sebum (oil). The farther a character is from the skin, the less likely a dermatologist is to include it in the story. Their heroes are chosen from the typical doctor's bag: creams, pills, needles. The antagonists are the villains *du jour*: dirt and bacteria. Dermatologists draw on statistics from the stage as they set it: "85 percent of people between the ages of 12 and 24 experience acne."[2] Is that 85 percent of young people everywhere, or 85 percent of certain young people from a certain time and place?

Another major voice in the acne story is the commercial skincare industry. Together with dermatologists, they are busy researching products and treatments to cure acne and capture a portion of the $120 billion global skincare market. But for a treatment to be profitable, it must be capable of being bottled and sold or administered in a doctor's office. The standards are even higher for the biggest source of funding in acne research, the pharmaceutical industry. If it can't be patented, what's the point?

But what if the cure for acne cannot be bottled, sold, administered or patented? Would we ever find it? If the main characters are not present on the surface of the skin or even listed on an ingredient label, would we ever notice them?

*****

---

[2] This statistic is from the American Academy of Dermatology's online "Stats and Facts" for acne. To receive a .pdf file with links to the online references discussed in this book, visit **ProjectFree.Me/References.**

The (Partial) Story of Me

I am not a dermatologist, an esthetician, a nutritionist or any other type of health professional. I'm an intelligence specialist at the Federal Bureau of Investigation (FBI) in Washington, D.C. You might think I am an unlikely author for a book on acne, but looking back at my career and educational experiences I now realize they were perfectly tailored to solve a case like this one.

As an undergraduate student at Georgetown University, I majored in *Science, Technology, and International Affairs*. I am intrigued by the ways we choose to develop our scientific understanding, why certain ideas take hold and others do not, and how the repercussions of scientific advancements are felt on a global scale. I pursued a career in intelligence because, as a young college student in the late 1990s, I looked around at the world and saw terrorism as the biggest upcoming threat to our wellbeing.

After graduation, I entered the United States Navy and later transitioned to the Federal Bureau of Investigation as an intelligence analyst. During my time at the FBI, I was selected to be a Fulbright scholar at the University of St. Andrews in the United Kingdom where I worked as a research assistant to Dr. Alex Schmid, former head of the Terrorism Prevention Branch of the United Nations. At St. Andrews, I specialized in a branch of International Studies called Constructivism which involves uncovering hidden assumptions and exploring alternative scenarios through the deconstruction of discourse and linguistics—the analysis of stories.

After completing my graduate degree in Scotland, I was offered a position at The Boeing Company in Washington, D.C. Most people think of Boeing as an airplane manufacturer, but it also has an Intelligence and Analytics branch. At Boeing I was contracted to work full-time at FBI where I instruct an intelligence class at Quantico and travel throughout the country providing analytical support for FBI cases.

My area of expertise is helping investigators uncover critical information by assisting them in asking questions. Intelligence analysis involves more than just collecting "the facts" and assembling them into a finished product. People tend to think of analysis as a puzzle, but it is more like trying to assemble a puzzle when half the pieces are missing. Additionally, for reasons that may or may not be malicious in nature, someone mixed in pieces designed to look like they belong to your puzzle when they actually do not. Plus there is no picture on top of the box to guide your efforts.

Whether analyzing the cause of acne or the extent of a terrorist threat, the challenges of thoughtful analysis are substantial. One of the main reasons intelligence analysis is so difficult is because it deals with ambiguous and incomplete data. When we are confronted with inadequate information, we rely on certain subconscious mental processes to interpret it. We want to believe our thinking is guided by rationality and logic, but studies of psychology (and history) show otherwise. The human brain relies not on fact but on mental models— a type of story we tell ourselves—to make sense of the world. These models are essential in the functioning of our daily lives, but they also lead to common cognitive pitfalls. Professional analysts spend their careers trying to develop skill sets to help avoid these analytic traps. We never fully succeed, but gains can be made in trying.

In *Psychology of Intelligence Analysis*, a foundational work in the field, CIA veteran Dick Heuer explains one of the most fundamental principles of perception that affects analysis: "We tend to perceive what we expect to perceive."[3] This basic tenet of analytic theory is well known, and still we are surprised when we catch it in action, especially in ourselves.

Perhaps the most famous such experiment was conducted by Christopher Chabris and Daniel Simons. If you are unfamiliar with their work, you might find it worthwhile to participate in the

---

[3] Notice he says we see what we *expect* to see, not what we *want* to see. Heuer, Richards. *Psychology of Intelligence Analysis.* CIA Center for the Study of Analysis.

experiment yourself by viewing their 90-second video at ProjectFree.Me/Basketball. (But do it now without reading a single word further or else your results will be skewed. Go ahead, I'll wait...) The experiment shows that half of the thousands of people tasked to count the number of passes in a basketball video fail to notice a person in a gorilla suit walking across the middle of the stage and beating his fists on his chest. People who miss seeing the gorilla insist it was not there when they are told about it afterwards. As psychologist Daniel Kahneman explains, the gorilla study illustrates two important points about our minds: "we can be blind to the obvious, and we are also blind to our blindness."

In writing *The End of Acne*, my hope is to make apparent the invisible gorilla on the stage. Once you know to look for him, he is difficult to miss. After struggling with cystic acne for over twenty years, sometimes I wonder myself why it took me so long to put the pieces together. But hindsight is its own type of bias.

Some people might dismiss my experience with acne as anecdotal or balk at the idea of a health book written by a non-medical professional. My response to such notions are best illustrated with a story.

*****

Engineers and Anecdotes: A Love Story

Samuel P. Langley should have invented the airplane. He held an assistantship at the Harvard College Observatory, taught mathematics at the United States Naval Academy, was a frequent guest at the White House, and was named Secretary of the Smithsonian Institute in 1887. In an effort to create the world's first manned flying machine, Dr. Langley spent a decade studying the fledgling field of aeronautics research before receiving a grant of

$50,000 from the War Department to develop his Aerodrome design. It was the largest research project ever funded by the department at the time. Dr. Langley had access to the top scientists in the world and the latest technical research. He had hefty financial backing and the full support of the United States government (does this story sound familiar?). Yet after seventeen years of effort, Langley was unable to figure out one little detail: how to make the darn thing fly.

Orville and Wilbur Wright, on the other hand, had no such competitive advantages. Neither brother had a college education. Technically, they didn't even have high school diplomas. They funded their interest in flying machines with proceeds from their bicycle shop while working to build the world's first airplane as a hobby in their spare time. When they wanted information on the latest aeronautics research, their best option was to send a written request to the government via the U.S. Postal Service and hope for a helpful response. Unlike Dr. Langley, they weren't even able to bounce ideas off their best friend, Alexander Graham Bell, when they ran into a particularly vexing design challenge.

Yet on December 17, 1903, with the media and all esteemed aeronautical experts noticeably lacking in attendance, the Wright brothers' manned flying machine flew for 59 seconds over the dunes at Kitty Hawk. It took the Wright brothers just four years to create the Wright Flyer, but it took the U.S. government nearly 40 years to admit the Wright Flyer, and not Langley's Aerodrome, was the first manned, powered aircraft capable of flight.

In his bestselling book *Mastery*, Robert Greene explains why the Wright brothers succeeded while Samuel Langley and the U.S. government failed. Langley's team was composed of specialists focused on making the most efficient parts. The most powerful engine. The most aerodynamic wings. They had an expert military pilot, too. This kind of specialization meant the person who designed the wings was different than the person who tested them in the air. Each crew member knew their specialty, but they could only think about how all the parts fit together in abstract terms. In contrast, the Wright brothers personally designed their machine, built it, flew it, crashed it, picked up the pieces, and designed it again. This process allowed them to rapidly uncover flaws in their design and ways to work them out. As Greene states, "it gave them a *feel* for the product that could never be had in the abstract."

Hopefully the analogy I am drawing between the discovery of the airplane and the cure for acne is starting to become clear. In our story about the birth of aviation (and yes, there are other versions of the story where other flying machines flew first), we see how the Wright brothers' approach was successful because it merged aeronautical theory with the physical world in a way Langley's approach did not. This same approach can be applied to the problem of acne. Greene concludes, "Whatever you are creating or designing, you must test and use it yourself. Separating out the work will make you lose touch with its functionality." The Wright brothers understood their flying machine from the inside out. It wasn't just something they designed and built. It was something they *experienced*.

The experience of acne is wholly lacking in acne research. Individual accounts are dismissed as anecdotal (in a pejorative sense) and not worthy of consideration in serious study of the subject. Instead of mining anecdotal evidence for clues, acne researchers are preoccupied with producing expensive double-blind, placebo-controlled, randomized trials of prescribable treatments for publication in peer-reviewed journals. Or they focus on statistical analysis of epidemiological surveys that confuse correlation with causation and overlook nuanced complexities inherent in the study of the human body.

Engineers tend not to focus on this distinction between anecdotal and "science-based" evidence. When something seems to work in the real world, curiosity takes over and they tinker, test, and repeat until before they know it, they brought a new idea into being. No one told the Wright brothers their flying machine was anecdotal.

As someone who experiences acne, and not just studies it in the abstract, you have an advantage over the entire skincare industry in finding a cure. You can test your theories, make adjustments, and test them again at a pace the "experts" are incapable of matching. You know your test subject better than any outside researcher ever could; its history, its sensations, its environment are all intimately familiar to you. And because acne is something you experience, you will *feel* when you are onto something or when something is not right even before you identify the reason. In the story of acne, we are not the scientists. We are the engineers.

"Truth is what stands the test of experience."
—Albert Einstein

PART ONE: CAUSE (*n.*)

1

WHY KITAVAN ISLANDERS DON'T HAVE ACNE, BUT AMERICANS DO

BY THE TIME THE SOCIETY FOR INVESTIGATIVE DERMATOLOGY held its 65th annual meeting in April 2004, they were certain they had the connection between diet and acne long figured out: there was none.

The persistent myth amongst laymen that acne is caused by what you eat was dispelled by science over thirty years prior. Its foundation began to crumble in 1969 when a clever dermatologist decided to give 65 subjects one candy bar per day for four weeks.[1] Half the subjects received candy bars with chocolate, but the candy bars provided to the other half of the subjects did not contain any chocolate at all. After four weeks, researchers did not notice any difference in the amount of acne developed by subjects in the two groups. It was damning evidence for the acne-diet proposition.

Just two years later, a study of 27 medical students provided all the affirmation dermatologists would need to abandon the unprofitable idea that acne is caused by diet.[2] The students were asked to identify the single food that was the most likely cause of their acne. It was a multiple-choice question and the possible answers were: (1) chocolate candy bars, (2) peanuts, (3) milk, or (4) Coca-Cola™. Each

---

[1] Fulton, J.E.; Plewig, G.; Kligman, A.M., "Effect of chocolate on acne vulgaris." *Journal of the American Medical Association.* 210:2071-2074, 1969.

[2] Anderson, P.C., "Foods as the cause of acne." *American Journal of Family Practitioners.* 3:102-103, 1971.

student was then given their suspected culprit food every day for one week. The dermatologist who conducted the study carefully counted and measured the acne lesions on each student before the study began and subsequently on each day of the study as students consumed their particular trigger food. At week's end again the results were clear. Diet does not cause acne.

For the next 34 years, not a single acne study was published examining the role of diet. In 2002, a comprehensive review of the scientific literature published on acne during the second half of the twentieth century revealed 99.6 percent of all acne studies failed to even mention diet, let alone study it as a potential cause of the disorder which affects millions of people each year.[3] This was the prevailing sentiment in April 2004 when the aforementioned Society for Investigative Dermatology invited a non-dermatologist, Dr. Loren Cordain, to speak at their 65th annual meeting.

Despite the title of doctor preceding his name, Cordain was likely the only one in the auditorium that evening without a degree in medicine. He was an exercise physiologist at Colorado State University with a specialty in evolutionary anthropology.

*****

Somewhere Over the Rainbow

Loren Cordain was inspired to apply his knowledge of evolutionary nutrition to the study of acne after reading an obscure article written by Otto Schaefer, a frontier physician who treated the Inuit people in the Arctic for 30 years in the mid twentieth century. The article, entitled "When the Eskimo Comes to Town," describes the decline in health that occurred when the Inuit people abandoned their

---

[3] Lehmann, H.P. et al, "Acne therapy: a methodologic review." *Journal of the American Academy of Dermatology.* 47:231-240, 2002.

traditional diet for modern foods.[4] Acne used to be unknown among Eskimos, but by the time Schaefer published his article in 1971, the change was readily apparent on the faces of Eskimo teenagers. Schaefer states, "One wonders what these people and the other old Northerners would think if they were to read some recent medical publications in which dermatologists belittle or deny the role of dietary factors in the pathogenesis of acne vulgaris."

Intrigued by Schaefer's account of the Eskimo, Cordain searched the scientific literature for more information on how acne is affected by diet and quickly noticed the dearth of research on the topic. He set out to study contemporary non-industrialized societies who, like the early Inuit, do not experience acne. His inquiry led to Kitava, one of the four major islands in the remote Trobriand Islands of Papua New Guinea in the Southwest Pacific. Approximately 2,250 native Kitavans lived on the island at the time, all without access to telephones, cars, or electricity. They subsisted primarily on a diet of fish, tubers, fruit, and coconut.

Staffan Lindeberg, a Swedish medical doctor and professor at the University of Lund, had been studying Kitavan Islanders since 1989 and found they did not experience diabetes, hypertension, heart disease, obesity, strokes, or acne. During a 7-week period in 1990, Lindeberg visited all 494 houses in Kitava and examined 1,200 Kitavans aged ten and older for skin disorders on their face and neck, and for males, on their back and chest as well. He did not find a single sign of acne in the entire population, including 300 teenagers and young adults between the ages of 15 and 25.

Other researchers observed a similar account with the Ache hunter-gatherers of eastern Paraguay whose traditional diet consisted mainly of wild and foraged foods and select cultivated crops such as manioc, maize, peanuts, and rice. As with the Kitavans, chronic disease including diabetes, asthma, hypertension, and other cardiovascular disease were rare among the Ache people. To determine

---

[4] Schaefer, O., "When the Eskimo comes to town." *Nutrition Today.* 6:8-16, 1971.

if they also did not exhibit acne, Cordain's co-researchers observed 115 Ache people over an 843-day period. Not a single case of acne was observed by any of the seven examining physicians throughout the length of the study.

Cordain and his colleagues published the results of their research in the 2002 *Archives of Dermatology* with the bold title, "Acne Vulgaris: A Disease of Western Civilization."[5] This was the topic of Cordain's presentation at the Society of Investigative Dermatology's annual meeting two years later. For over an hour, he explained the details of his theory which held promise for clarifying the recent unexplained rise in adult acne, particularly among women.

In light of the new evidence from Kitava and Paraguay, Cordain reinterpreted the results of the famous 1969 chocolate bar study as two of the study's authors listened from the audience. *Of course* the study showed no difference in acne between the people who ate the candy bars that contained chocolate and the ones that did not, Cordain explained. Acne is not caused by chocolate. It is caused by *sugar*. Both types of candy bars contained sugar in equal amounts, so they caused acne in equal amounts.

After ruling out genetic factors, Cordain and his team concluded that the reason people in Kitavan and Ache societies do not experience acne is because of their low-glycemic diets. As the theory goes, when people eat high-glycemic foods (e.g., soft drinks, bread, sweets, pasta) their blood insulin levels spike and cause a series of hormonal events that increase the production of testosterone and other growth factors. This hormonal cascade stimulates the excess production of oil and an overgrowth of cells lining the pores, leading to inflammation and the bacterial infections that cause acne.

After Cordain completed his groundbreaking presentation, one of the authors of the chocolate study reached over and shook his hand.

---

[5] Cordain, L.; Lindeberg, S.; Hurtado, M., et al., "Acne vulgaris: a disease of western civilization." *Archives of Dermatology.* 138:1584-1590, 2002.

"Thank you for correcting our mistake," he said.[6]

Over the next few years, researchers published studies that Cordain would later refer to as "the trump card"—randomized controlled human trials that prove his theory on diet and acne is correct. When study participants consumed a low-glycemic diet, they exhibited a measurable decrease in acne lesions.[7] The proof was in the sugar-free pudding.

In 2006, Cordain authored a book called *The Dietary Cure for Acne* that outlines his anti-acne diet for the average reader and includes an entire chapter of unsolicited success stories. He also published numerous non-acne books on the dietary principles he uncovered in his research. Cordain started referring to his nutritional approach as the Paleo Diet with the launch of his book by the same name in 2002. He went on to be known as the father of the paleo movement, one of the most popular health movements of the early twenty-first century.

Cordain and his colleagues believed they identified the "holy grail" of acne research. Dermatologists long understood the proximate causes of acne—blocked pores, excess oil, bacteria, and inflammation—but the ultimate cause of acne was admittedly elusive.

---

[6] Oaklander, Mandy. "The New Science of Clear Skin." *Prevention.* May 13, 2014.

[7] Smith, R.N.; Mann, N.J.; Mäkeläinen, H.; Roper, J.; Braue ,A.; Varigos, G., "A pilot study to determine the short-term effects of a low glycemic load diet on hormonal markers of acne: a nonrandomized, parallel, controlled feeding trial." *Molecular Nutrition and Food Research.* 52(6):718-726, 2008.

Smith, R.N.; Braue, A.; Varigos, G.A.; Mann, N.J., "The effect of a low glycemic load diet on acne vulgaris and the fatty acid composition of skin surface triglycerides." *Journal of Dermatological Science.* 50(1):41-52, 2008.

Smith, R.N.; Mann, N.J.; Braue, A.; Mäkeläinen, H.; Varigos, G.A., "A low-glycemic-load diet improves symptoms in acne vulgaris patients: a randomized controlled trial." *American Journal of Clinical Nutrition.* 86(1):107-115, 2007.

Smith, R.N.; Mann, N.J.; Braue, A.; Mäkeläinen, H.; Varigos, G.A., "The effect of a high-protein, low glycemic-load diet versus a conventional, high glycemic-load diet on biochemical parameters associated with acne vulgaris: a randomized, investigator-masked, controlled trial." *Journal of the American Academy of Dermatology.* 57(2): 247-256, 2007.

Cordain's insulin theory showed the root cause of acne is high-glycemic foods. There was just one gorilla-ish problem. In the human trials his associates conducted, acne lesions were observably lessened, but they did not disappear altogether. Likewise, the chapter of testimonials in Cordain's acne book is brimming with phrases like "significantly reduced" and "a big improvement." One person even writes "my acne ALMOST cleared up" two times in his testimonial when he tried to implement the paleo diet on two separate occasions.

Dermatologist Susan Bershad responded to Cordain's article in the *Archives of Dermatology* with an article of her own entitled, "The Unwelcome Return of the Acne Diet."[8] She points out that some American teens who are not inclined to eat sweets or drink soft drinks consume a relatively low glycemic load yet are still prone to acne.

Was this another instance of a dermatologist's subconscious effort to preserve the future of her profession by sabotaging scientific evidence that diet causes acne? Perhaps, but she had a point.

*****

Gorilla in the Mist

When Cordain's team published their revolutionary paper in 2002 asserting acne is a disease of western civilization, I was somewhere in the Atlantic Ocean oblivious of the scientific literature on acne and yet busy conducting experiments of my own on a sample size of one. But to know the full story, we need to rewind to a few years earlier.

From my adolescence in suburban America to Scotland, the edge of the Sahara, and even months at sea, each of these places offered clues that would later prove instrumental in solving the acne

---

[8] Bershad, Susan. "The Unwelcome Return of the Acne Diet," *Archives of Dermatology,* 139(7):940-941, 2003.

mystery. If you read the story carefully, you will see the gorilla enter stage left and exit stage right no less than *four* times. He even beats his fists on his chest once or twice. See if you can spot him.

Looking back over my experience with acne, it would be difficult to remember when I had it and when I didn't if not for a few bookmarks along the way. I'm sure you know what I mean. The miracle treatment that worked for a while and then somehow stopped working. The unexpected side effects. The flareups so sudden and overwhelming you thought your face caught fire. The offhand comments that pierce thick skin but lodge in your memory.

During my adolescent years in the suburbs of Philadelphia, I didn't focus on my acne much. I would not even remember having acne in middle school if not for a particular conversation that stuck in my mind. I was walking back from lunch with a group of classmates when one of them said, "Can you believe Kelly never had a pimple?" The answer was no. I *couldn't* believe it. I remember looking at her in amazement and thinking, how is that possible? Clearly I must have had my fair share of acne already. I just assumed it was a part of life. (Cue the gorilla.)

After high school, I moved to Washington, D.C. to attend college at Georgetown. By the end of sophomore year, my skin was so bad that it was time to see a professional. My consultation with the dermatologist was a blur. I remember him bursting into the exam room, studying my face for a minute (maybe), and then saying a few words to my mother before speaking predominantly to his tape recorder. Even in such clinical terms, it sounded strange to hear someone talk about the placement and severity of my acne as if I were not in the room. Before leaving, the dermatologist handed my mother a prescription for Accutane and a topical treatment along with some cursory instructions. That was the last appointment I ever had with a dermatologist about my acne.

I started taking Accutane the summer before my junior year, which I spent abroad in Senegal, West Africa. After arriving in Senegal,

I grew increasingly concerned about the warning label on the bottle about avoiding sun exposure. How do I avoid the sun while living on the edge of the Sahara? My skin had already cleared up, so I took it upon myself to discontinue the medication soon after my arrival. I remained effortlessly free of acne for the rest of the year. I remember thinking, "Wow, Accutane works great!" But that was not the whole story.

After my junior year in Senegal, I travelled to Hawaii to spend a month on the *USS Carl Vinson* as part of my training as a Navy midshipman. Even though I had only been back in the U.S. for a few weeks before leaving for Hawaii, my skin had already returned to full blown acne mode. After reporting aboard, I visited the ship library to pick up some books to entertain me during my free time at sea. When I returned the books at the end of the month, the library custodian remarked, "Your skin really cleared up since the first time you came in." How do you respond to a statement like that. Thanks? But the jerk librarian was right. Why was it so easy to be acne-free on the ship?

Returning to Georgetown for senior year, my acne returned too. This time I decided to try Proactiv, a skincare system comprised of a daily cleanser, toner, moisturizer, and spot treatment along with a weekly mask to remove the impurities that remained. The active ingredients—mainly benzoyl peroxide, sulfur, and salicylic acid— helped keep my acne under control, but they were no match for what my face would face next.

When I moved to Rhode Island to start my navy career, within days my skin was the worst it had ever been. I had deep cystic welts on my chin, cheeks, forehead, even behind my ears and down my neck. I tried the Murad line. Then Dermalogica. Nothing provided relief. It burned even when I rinsed my face with plain tap water. I started to wonder if something in the water was aggravating my skin. I lived in a historic house in Newport; maybe the pipes were made of lead? I began using bottled water to wash my face and I thought it helped a little, but thankfully my time in Newport was short-lived.

After just six months in Rhode Island, I transferred to Norfolk, Virginia to report for my first assignment on the *USS Wasp*. I was hoping my skin would clear up on the *Wasp* like it did on the *Carl Vinson*, but no such luck. One day the ship's doc knocked on my door. "I noticed you have acne," he said. "I can write a prescription for that." I thanked him and politely declined even though I *should* have accused him of trying to mutilate my unborn children. Birth defects are just one of the documented side effects of acne medication.

I felt embarrassed by the doc's unsolicited offer. Apparently my acne was still a prominent feature. How was I supposed to establish my reputation as a respected navy officer as a five foot two female with a face full of pimples?

After my tour in Virginia, the Navy transferred me to Puerto Rico and then Jacksonville, Florida. In Puerto Rico my skin wasn't bad, but the acne returned in Jacksonville. I kept it under control through monthly facials (sometimes weekly) and the use of a common acne cleanser that contains high amounts of benzoyl peroxide—five times the amount found in the Proactiv line. It bleached the heck out of my towels but it was the only product that kept my acne in check.

At this point, I was nearing thirty. That is when my skin threw me a major curve ball. I just left Jacksonville to accept a Fulbright scholarship in Tunisia, another sun-soaked country on the edge of the Sahara. At the end of a day at the beach in Tunisia, I noticed a dark shadow on my upper lip. I thought it was a smudge of dirt but it wouldn't wipe off. I looked at the mirror again. What was it? I felt my stomach tighten. Is this what skin cancer looks like? Is it permanent? Will it spread? As if looking like mini-Hitler wasn't bad enough.

The dark patch of skin turned out to be melasma, a common skin condition triggered by sun exposure. After researching melasma on the internet, I saw that some people drew a connection between the use of benzoyl peroxide and the onset of their melasma. I stopped using benzoyl peroxide and my melasma went away. The strange part was that my acne didn't come back, either.

I spent the second part of my Fulbright studies in Scotland where, like in Tunisia, my skin was effortlessly clear. While in Scotland, I turned thirty and had a cellulite-fueled health awakening after a cliché encounter with a dressing room mirror. I cleaned up my diet and rid my apartment of toxic products. I ate wild salmon, switched to herbal tea, and started using fluoride-free toothpaste. The only time I had acne was when I broke my routine and travelled away from my little flat in St. Andrews. I remember telling a friend, "It took some work but at thirty years old, I finally figured out how to get rid of my acne."

Not yet, Melissa.

*****

Once Upon a Dream

After Scotland, I returned to the United States to live in Delray Beach near Miami, Florida. My acne returned quickly and was the worst it had been since I lived in Newport, Rhode Island.[9] It became so bad, I resorted to using benzoyl peroxide again, but then the melasma came back, too.

I developed deep cystic welts around my mouth, along my jawline, forehead, down the front and back of my neck, and even inside my ears. I could feel each breakout forming a week before it came to the surface, erupting in a tender white volcano that took another two weeks to heal. This time, with my health awakening firmly entrenched, I looked to alternative treatments to heal my skin. I used apple cider vinegar as a toner and coconut oil as a moisturizer. I coated my face in clay. I took evening primrose oil and probiotics. I went for acupuncture. I did yoga.

---

[9] For the ugly photographic evidence, see ProjectFree.Me/The-End-of-Acne.

One night my acne was bothering me so much I couldn't sleep. I wandered downstairs to the refrigerator, desperate for relief. Lying on the couch, I gently painted my skin with yogurt. Its coldness was the only comfort I could think of for the mass of inflammation formerly known as my face. *Acne was driving me mad.*

Why after all these years was I still struggling with acne? Why do I have acne even though I take meticulous care of my skin? How do people who eat nothing but junk food *not* have acne, but I do? I could not figure it out. I was defeated. Yogurt tears dripped down my face.

I needed professional help but traditional doctors had proven useless in the past. During a required annual physical with the Navy, one doctor suggested to heal my acne I should (1) stop touching my face with my hands, (2) clean telephone receivers before making phone calls, and (3) take a multi-vitamin. This kind of advice from physicians was insulting but typical. Clearly my skin problem was more complicated than that. They did not know me well enough to realize how ridiculous their suggestions sounded. They did not know me, or my acne story, at all.

Because of my interest in studying cellulite, I started to read about the lymphatic system and its effect on health. The lymphatic system consists of a series of nodes and vessels that circulate fluid called lymph from the tissues to the bloodstream. I decided to consult a lymph drainage specialist to see if it would help with my acne. I was fortunate to live near the Upledger Institute, one of the preeminent facilities in the world for Lymph Drainage Therapy, a light-touch therapy created by French physician Bruno Chikly. The therapist I consulted, Mya Breman, studied closely with Dr. Chikly and was a longtime practitioner at Upledger.

After each session with Mya, I noticed immediate improvement. The redness and swelling decreased overnight. Existing blemishes healed at an astounding rate. But within two to three days, my skin would return to its normal distressed state. After a few weeks of treatment, Mya suggested I take a break from our sessions until I could figure out what was causing the breakouts in the first place. Mya is a Licensed Clinical Social Worker and at our last session, she decided to make use of her psychotherapy training to help me get to the root of the problem.

"If your acne was a cartoon character," Mya asked, "what would it look like?"

I thought the question was silly but I followed her instructions and said the first thing that came to mind. "If my acne was a cartoon character, it would be an oil drop."

"When did this oil drop form?" she asked.

"Seventh grade," I responded.

"Are you sure it hasn't been around longer than that?" Mya asked. In true psychotherapy style, I was soon answering questions about my deepest childhood fears. I continued to respond with the first thing that popped into my mind. I was *most* afraid of the dentist. I laughed at first, but then realized how real the fear was as a child. One year, my dentist required the extraction of four of my baby teeth. Each tooth made a cracking sound I can still hear today as it loosened from my jaw. I was seven. My mom said I was such a good little girl for the dentist and didn't even cry until the car ride on the way home.

I continued to ponder this unearthed childhood fear over the next few days. I thought of all the other things I hated about going to the dentist. The drooling. The scraping. The needles in places there should *not* be needles. The feeling of vulnerability lying in the dentist's chair. The awkward fluoride trays. As a child, my dentist directed my parents to give me fluoride pills, which I later learned are the reason my teeth are slightly discolored. It's a condition called dental fluorosis and a common indicator of fluoride toxicity.[10]

One night after my last session with Mya, I had a dream about going to the dentist. I was a small child again in the dentist's chair. There was a fluoride tray in my mouth but this time the tray was made

---

[10] Whitford, G.M., "The physiological and toxicological characteristics of fluoride." *Journal of Dental Research.* 69: 539-549, 1990.

of glass. When the dentist tried to remove it, the tray shattered into a thousand pieces embedding small shards of glass deep in my gums. My subconscious already knew.

I remember exactly where I was standing when the idea first struck my conscious mind. I was visiting my boyfriend's family in central Florida for Thanksgiving when I was explaining my frustration with acne to his sister, a physician. There was a glass of tap water in my hand and I was about to take a sip. I looked at the water and the idea came to me: maybe my cystic acne was caused by drinking fluoride.

I was aware that fluoride could cause acne through topical contact,[11] a condition known as fluoroderma.[12] From the *Physician's Desk Reference*: "In hypersensitive individuals, fluorides occasionally cause skin eruptions such as atopic dermatitis... These hypersensitivity reactions usually disappear promptly after discontinuation of the fluoride."[13] But I washed my face with bottled water and used non-fluoridated toothpaste. The idea did not occur to me until precisely that moment that perhaps cystic acne could be caused by fluoride *ingestion*. Multiple case studies from the 1960s and 1970s indicate that fluoride ingestion can cause skin conditions such as dermatitis, eczema, and hives.[14] Could fluoride cause cystic acne, too?

I did a quick internet search to see if my current residence was fluoridated. It was, and the amount was towards the upper limit of the Center for Disease Control's recommended upper guideline of 1.2 milligrams per liter. The last time my skin was this bad was when I

---

[11] Saunders, M.A., "Fluoride Toothpaste: A Cause of Acne-like Eruptions." *Archives of Dermatology.* 111:793, 1975.

[12] Blasik, L.G.; Spencer, S.K., "Fluoroderma." *Archives of Dermatology.* 115(11); 1334-1335, 1979.

[13] *Physician's Desk Reference*, 48:2335-2338, 1994.

[14] Feltman, R.; Kosel, G., "Prenatal and postnatal ingestion of fluorides - Fourteen years of investigation - Final report." *Journal of Dental Medicine.* 16:190-199, 1969.

Shea, J.J.; Gillespie, S.M.; Waldbott, G.L., "Allergy to fluoride." *Annals of Allergy.* 25:388-391, 1969.

lived in Newport, Rhode Island. Do they fluoridate there? Yes. Not only that, but when I visited the Newport water municipality website, they happened to be displaying a notice to consumers informing them that a random spot test indicated they accidentally added too much fluoride to the water—over twice the upper recommended amount—and it would take some time before it returned to recommended levels. I wondered how often they accidentally over-fluoridate their population.

The whole story of my experience with acne flashed in front of me. Philadelphia, Washington, D.C., Norfolk, and Jacksonville are all fluoridated. Senegal, Puerto Rico, Tunisia, and Scotland are not. The *USS Carl Vinson* uses reverse osmosis to purify water at sea. The *Wasp* took on fluoridated water from the Norfolk Naval Station. The only time I had breakouts in Scotland was when I travelled overnight outside of St. Andrews. My toiletry bag held a small travel tube of fluoridated toothpaste.

It all made sense. My dream about the fluoride tray. My fear of dentists—my acne was caused by consuming *fluoride* and my deepest self knew it.

If anecdotal evidence is ignored in studies of acne, what do you think the medical community would say about hypotheses received through dreams and epiphanies? But the fact that the idea of fluoride-induced acne came to me this way should not be surprising. There is a long history of scientific advancements first conceived in dreams.[15] In his bestselling book, *The Myths of Innovation,* Scott Berkun claims the experience of epiphany is misunderstood. As with the famous story of Isaac Newtown discovering the law of gravity when an apple fell on his head, people mistake epiphanies for haphazard ideas when they are actually the culmination of years of careful inquiry—the piece of a puzzle that brings the full picture into view.

As Berkun explains, epiphanies are preceded by a long period

---

[15] For some examples, see Kuhn, Thomas. *The Structure of Scientific Revolutions.* 4th ed. Chicago: The University of Chicago Press, 2012, p. 122.

spent understanding the problem and immersing oneself in the domain (my history with acne). Then there is a period of incubation during which the knowledge is digested and rough attempts at solutions are made (my experiments with acne treatments). Sometimes, as Berkun points out, there are long pauses during incubation when progress stalls and confidence wanes (my yogurt tears).

But then the big insights, if they occur, happen in the depths of incubation. Berkun explains, "It's possible these pauses are minds catching up with everything they've observed" (my dream about the fluoride tray). He concludes, "When a promising idea surfaces out of the subconscious and rises into our active minds, it can feel like it came from somewhere else because we weren't aware of our subconscious thoughts while we were mowing the lawn." Or drinking a glass of water.

Over the next few years, I put my fluoride theory to the test of experience. Unfortunately it is not a simple matter of drinking bottled water. Fluoride is insidious in the industrialized diet. It hides in food and beverages where you would never find it if you did not know to look. But whenever I had an acne flareup, I was able to use the scientific literature to track it back to a few hours earlier when I consumed food or beverages that contained a significant amount of fluoride. This happened every time, without exception. In this way, my cystic acne served as a guide that helped me figure out how to limit my fluoride consumption and ultimately cure my chronic acne.

It was a strange coincidence, if you believe in that sort of thing, that my fluoride epiphany occurred in Polk County. Located in central Florida, Polk County is the heart of the U.S. phosphate industry. Prior to World War II, the area was known for its livestock and citrus cultivation, but after the war over a dozen phosphate plants were established there to process phosphate ore for the production of commercial fertilizer.

In the 1950s, unchecked pollution from the newly constructed phosphate plants released large quantities of fluoride into the atmosphere.[16] Raw phosphate ore is roughly two to four percent fluoride. It was absorbed by nearby vegetation, damaging 25,000 acres of citrus crops and causing mass poisoning of grazing cattle. In the words of the former President of the Polk County Cattleman's Association, "We watched our cattle become gaunt and starved, their legs became deformed; they lost their teeth. Reproduction fell off and when a cow did have a calf, it was also affected by this malady or was a stillborn."[17] An estimated 30,000 cattle were lost and 150,000 acres of grazing land were abandoned.

The Environmental Protection Agency (EPA) now requires "wet scrubbers" to be installed on all phosphate processing plants to capture smokestack pollution before it enters the air. *This unfiltered pollution is then barreled and sold as fluoride to our municipal water authorities for addition to public water supplies.*

Most Americans, if we think about such matters, assume the fluoride added to the public water supply is a pharmaceutical grade fluoride like the kind used in toothpaste and mouthwash, or in government studies of the safety of fluoridation. This is not the case. Approximately 95 percent of the fluoride used for public water fluoridation in the United States is hydrofluorosilicic acid, an *unfiltered* byproduct of the phosphate fertilizer industry.[18]

I found this fact difficult to believe until I saw it in writing on my own local municipality's annual water quality report. Next to the

---

[16] Connett, Michael. "The Phosphate Industry: An Environmental Overview," May 2003 (available at www.fluoridealert.org/articles/phosphate01/).

[17] Linton, Ron, *Terracide: America's Destruction of Her Living Environment.* Little Brown & Company, 1970 (as cited at www.fluoridealert.org/phosphate/overview.htm).

[18] "Water Fluoridation Additives Fact Sheet," Center for Disease Control (available at www.cdc.gov/fluoridation/factsheets/engineering/wfadditives.htm). Also see "Fluoridation Chemicals" by the Fluoride Action Network for more information on industrial sources of fluoride used in water fluoridation and issues concerning lead and arsenic contamination (available at www.fluoridealert.org/issues/water/fluoridation-chemicals/).

line where the amount of fluoride was measured within "recommended" levels is a note: "discharges from fertilizer and aluminum factories." This discharge from commercial fertilizer plants is sold to water municipalities throughout the United States and Canada, including towns near you and ones as far north as the Arctic.

*****

A Galaxy Far, Far Away

In *The Dietary Cure for Acne*, Loren Cordain, founder of the modern paleo movement and outspoken critic of the industrialized diet, does not account for fluoride in his assessment of acne. He is so focused on the leading actors in his story of heart disease (e.g., sugar, carbs, insulin, inflammation) that he completely overlooks fluoride, a hidden but pervasive element of industrialized life.

Cordain's research philosophy provides foreshadowing that things are about to go wrong. His self-described motto, "Let the data speak for itself,"[19] is an impossibility. Data does not speak. As with intelligence analysis, scientific facts require a translator, someone to put the facts into language and tell their story to the world. The studies that uncover the facts require a designer, someone to decide which variables are important and which are not, which parameters will be accounted for and which will not. The analyst's voice cannot be removed from the data. When we fool ourselves into thinking otherwise, grave errors are to be expected.

Cordain points to the controlled human trials conducted by Neil Mann and his colleagues at RMIT University in Australia as proof that a high glycemic diet causes acne. But looking at his trump card

---

[19] See "Exclusive interview with Godfather of Paleo Loren Cordain!" by Paleo Cafe, July 24, 2015 (available at http://paleo-cafe.com.au/2015/07/exclusive-interview-paleo-founder-loren-cordain/).

through the lens of the fluoride theory, a clearer picture comes into focus. In Mann's 2007 study published in the *American Journal of Clinical Nutrition,* 43 males between the ages of 15 and 25 were divided into two groups.[20] One group consumed a low glycemic load (LGL) diet with foods high in protein and complex carbohydrates. The other group consumed a high glycemic load diet (HGL) composed of carbohydrate-dense foods they typically ate in their regular lives. At the end of the 12-week study, researchers counted the number of acne lesions and, as expected, found a marked decrease in the group on the low glycemic diet.

The authors of the study provide few details on the composition of the HGL and LGL diets beyond the ratio of carbs, fat and protein, but in similar studies published a few months later by the same researchers, they include a table to illustrate the types of foods consumed by participants in each group.[21] In addition to other foods, both groups consumed water, low-fat milk, cereals, juice, and different types of rice. Any of these foods can contain significant amounts of fluoride. But the breakfast cereals consumed by the LGL group were whole grain while the control group was given extruded corn, rice, or wheat -based cereals. As you will learn in chapter four, extruded cereals processed in fluoridated water have been found to contain fluoride concentrations between 3.8 and 6.3 parts per million (ppm), an amount several times higher than the 0.7 ppm dose currently

---

[20] Smith, R.N.; Mann, N.J.; Braue, A.; Mäkeläinen, H.; Varigos, G.A., "A low-glycemic-load diet improves symptoms in acne vulgaris patients: a randomized controlled trial." *American Journal of Clinical Nutrition.* 86(1):107-115, 2007.

[21] Smith, R.; Mann, N.; Mäkeläinen, H.; Roper, J.; Braue, A.; Varigos, G., "A pilot study to determine the short-term effects of a low glycemic load diet on hormonal markers of acne: a nonrandomized, parallel, controlled feeding trial." *Molecular Nutrition and Food Research.* 52(6):718-726, 2008.

Smith, R.N.; Braue, A.; Varigos, G.A.; Mann, N.J., "The effect of a low glycemic load diet on acne vulgaris and the fatty acid composition of skin surface triglycerides." *Journal of Dermatological Science.* 50(1):41-52, 2008.

recommended by dental authorities in the United States.[22] The muesli and whole oats consumed by the LGL group in Mann's studies likely did not contain significant amounts of fluoride.

Another nuanced difference between the diets was the type of juice the participants were provided. The LGL group was given apple juice while the HGL group drank orange juice. We are not told the brands of juice but it is probable they varied widely in their fluoride content. Researchers at Tufts University measured 43 varieties of juice and found a range of fluoride between 0.15 and 6.8 ppm.[23] Apple juice is often 100 percent juice while orange juice tends to be made from concentrate with fluoridated water. The pesticide load of the fruit also contributes to the overall fluoride content.

Furthermore, the HGL group was allowed orange-flavored soft drinks and cordial beverages, two more potential caloric sources of fluoride. Only subjects in the HGL group were allowed to eat potatoes. Were they fried and roasted—or boiled and mashed in fluoridated water? The study was conducted in the fluoridated city of Melbourne, Australia.

Looking at this study through fluoride-colored glasses, it becomes clear the research team and their randomized controlled trials were no match for the insidious nature of a culprit like fluoride. Cordain frequently refers to the study's author as Neil Mann, a fellow professor and nutritional biochemist at RMIT University. But the primary author on all three publications cited above is listed as Robyn Smith, a postgraduate scholar funded by the National Meat Industry Training Council of Australia. I am not implying that Smith consciously influenced the study to prove a low glycemic, high protein diet is beneficial for acne. But it is not a coincidence the results were good for business.

------

[22] Warren, J.J.; Levy, S.M., "Current and future role of fluoride in nutrition." *Dental Clinics of North America*, 47: 225-243, 2003.

[23] Stannard, J.G., et al., "Fluoride levels and fluoride contamination of fruit juices." *Journal of Clinical Pediatric Dentistry.* 16(1):38-40, 1991.

In his bestselling book *Influence*, Robert Cialdini describes the number one principle of persuasion: reciprocation. Even when given an inconsequential gift or favor, a powerful human drive kicks in and compels us to return the favor—and with interest. Sociologists have not found a single human society that does not subscribe to the rule of reciprocity, making it illogical (and unscientific) to assume the scientific results of scientific research are not skewed by the source of science funding.

Famed archaeologist Richard Leakey described the principle of reciprocity as the essence of what it means to be human. To quote Leakey, "We are human because our ancestors learned to share their food and their skills in an honored network of obligation." The power of reciprocity is so overwhelming that we are *obligated* to comply even when the gift is unwanted, let alone when it covers research costs and tuition for graduate school. Smith and Mann's studies note that "Meat and Livestock Australia had no role in data collection, data analysis, data interpretation, or submission for publication."[24] But when industry helped write the screenplay and then held casting calls for the main actors, the gorilla was not invited to audition.

To be clear, I am not arguing there are no health benefits for the paleo diet, even specifically for healing acne. As Cordain's success stories show, the paleo diet can be widely effective at reducing acne—just not for the reasons he thinks it is. To implement the diet, Cordain advises to restrict consumption of many of the potentially high-fluoride foods commonly consumed today, such as cereal, soft drinks, rice, pasta, potatoes, beans, canned fish and meats, milk, beer, wine, and other alcoholic beverages. He even recommends avoiding dates and raisins, two fruits that can cause fluoroderma flareups for reasons that will be explained later. (Don't worry, you won't have to eliminate all these foods from your diet to heal your acne. It will all make sense

---

[24] Smith, R.N.; Braue, A.; Varigos, G.A.; Mann, N.J., "The effect of a low glycemic load diet on acne vulgaris and the fatty acid composition of skin surface triglycerides." *Journal of Dermatological Science.* 50(1):41-52, 2008.

by the end of the book.) With so many items on the "do not consume" list, it is likely many paleo dieters will *almost* heal their acne. And this is exactly what their experience shows.

Cordain starts to lose his footing when he strays too far from the visible evidence he was seeing in the physical world—the lack of acne on Kitavan faces—and instead tumbles head-first into the abstract ideas manifest predominantly in the world of scientific discourse. His book on acne is filled with the stories of, for example, IL-1 alpha (Obe-Wan) labelled as cytokine (Jedi).[25] Then there are the keratinocytes (Anakin Skywalker) which eventually become corneocytes (Darth Vader) and prevent desmosomes (Palpatine) from disintegration.[26] And of course, IGF-1/IGFBP-3 (R2-D2 and C-3PO).[27]

When asked about his research methods following the findings in Kitava, Cordain explains, "What I had to do was go back into the dermatology/medical literature and back engineer the mechanism by which a western diet could elicit acne at the cellular level. I accomplished this by immersing myself in the salient literature to develop a hypothetical mechanism which was verified four years later by my colleague, Neil Mann."[28]

If instead of all that, Cordain simply limited his assessment to phenomenon he was observing in the physical world (using the force) instead of diving into the parallel galaxy of scientific parlance (the dark side), his article would have concluded that acne vulgaris is a

---

[25] "IL-1 alpha is a cell-to-cell messenger produced by white blood cells called monocytes. Because it is a localized hormone, it is labeled a 'cytokine'..." Cordain, *The Dietary Cure for Acne*, p 51.

[26] "As keratinocytes begin to turn into corneocytes, the molecular structure of the desmosomes starts to change...You also know that the reason why these corneocytes stick together is because their cell-to-cell anchors (the desmosomes) fail to disintegrate properly and on time." Cordain, *The Dietary Cure for Acne*, pp. 40/59.

[27] "One final note on the IGF-1/ IGFBP-3 story... the binding of IGF-1 to IGFBP-3 is not a good thing for acne sufferers because as with high glycemic load carbs, it, in effect, reduces IGFBP-3." Cordain, *The Dietary Cure for Acne*, p. 50.

[28] See "Dr. Pastore's Questions" (available at http://thepaleodiet.com/dr-pastores-qa-with-dr-cordain/).

disease of western civilization. Full stop. It would have brought dermatologists a giant step forward in their stated mission of identifying the ultimate cause of acne, without sending them into a wild Hoth asteroid field. (Sorry. No more Star Wars references. Promise.)

On further reading of Otto Schaefer's "When the Eskimo Comes to Town"—the article that sparked Cordain's interest in studying acne as a disease of western civilization—we see clues that fluoride played a starring role in the Inuit story. First, Schaefer makes clear the Eskimos with acne were the ones who "came to town," as the title of his article indicates. And not just any town. Eskimos with acne were seen predominantly on the streets of *larger* towns. Schaefer states, "The condition used to be unknown among Eskimos, but one can see it readily amongst teenagers on the streets of Inuvik, Frobisher Bay, and Cambridge Bay. It is far less prevalent in the smaller centers." And yes, dentists already brought their water fluoridation programs to larger towns in the Arctic at this time. Schaefer's article was written in 1971. Fluoridation began in Frobisher Bay six years earlier.[29] It was implemented in Inuvik in 1962.[30]

In addition to fluoride in the water, Eskimos were consuming fluoride hidden in other industrialized beverages. Cordain focuses on soft drinks because they contain sugar, but the imported soft drinks the Eskimos were drinking likely contained fluoride, as well, since they were mostly produced in urban centers where the water supply was fluoridated. Schaefer points out, "Many Eskimos themselves blame their pimples on the 'pop, chocolate, and candies' the youngsters consume as if addicted." In Arctic towns where drinking water was often brought in by truck, as was the case in Cambridge Bay, soft drinks offered a cheap alternative.

---

[29] Curzon, M.E.J.; Curzon, J.A., "Dental caries prevalence in the Baffin Island Eskimo." *Pediatric Dentistry*, 1(3), 1979.

[30] Email correspondence with Justin Hazenberg, Engineering Team Lead, Water and Sanitation for the Department of Municipal and Community Affairs, Government of the Northwest Territories, Oct 22, 2015.

Another possible way Inuit societies were suddenly exposed to increased levels of fluoride was through a longstanding and seemingly innocuous legacy of colonialism: black tea. Along with sugar and tobacco, tea was a popular commodity at fur trading posts throughout Canada and is the most consumed beverage in the world, next to water. It also contains more fluoride than any other edible plant. In a 2005 study published in the *American Journal of Medicine,* researchers measured some preparations of tea that contain fluoride at 6.5 ppm.[31] (The maximum contaminant level currently set by the EPA for drinking water is 4 ppm.) New research indicates the level of fluoride in tea could be even higher when using more comprehensive measuring methods.[32]

From countries as far spread as Chile,[33] China,[34] Senegal,[35] and Jordan,[36] to name just a few, studies show fluoride from tea consumption causes dental and skeletal fluorosis. In Lindeberg's study of Kitavan islanders, he notes their consumption of tea was "close to nil" which helps explain their complete lack of acne.[37] Likewise, the Ache people in Paraguay drink yerba tea which is derived from a species of the holly family, not the camellia sinensis plant from which

---

[31] Whyte, M.P.; Essmyer, K.; Gannon, F.H.; Reinus, W.R., "Skeletal fluorosis and instant tea." *American Journal of Medicine,* 118(1):78-82, 2005.

[32] Public release from the Medical College of Georgia, "Tea Contains More Fluoride Than Once Thought," Georgia Regents University, July 14, 2010.

[33] Sergio Gomez, S., et al., "Fluoride content of tea and amount ingested by children." *Odontologia Chilena,* 37(2):251-255, 1989.

[34] Cao, J., et al., "Brick tea consumption as the cause of dental fluorosis among children from Mongol, Kazak and Yugu populations in China." *Food and Chemical Toxicology.* 35(8):827-833, 1997.

[35] Diouf, A., et al., "Dietary intake of fluorine through use of tea prepared by the traditional method in Senegal." *Dakar Medical.* 39(2):227-230, 1994.

[36] Fraysse, C., et al., "The role of tea consumption in dental fluorosis in Jordan." *Bulletin du Groupement International pour la Recherche Scientifique en Stomatologie et Odontologie,* 32(1):39-46, 1989.

[37] Cordain, L.; Lindeberg, S.; Hurtado, M., et al., "Acne vulgaris: a disease of western civilization." *Archives of Dermatology.* 138:1584-1590, 2002.

common black tea is produced. Yerba tea is not a significant source of fluoride. I propose tea and other common sources of fluoride contributed to the sudden development of acne among the Eskimos in the 1960s and to the stratospheric rate of acne in our own society today —including yours.

We will return to the topic of dietary fluoride in an upcoming chapter. But first, if you associate fluoride with healthy smiles, and anti-fluoridationists with *Dr. Strangelove*, then you are likely missing a few key scenes in the fluoride story.[38] How could a naturally-occurring mineral touted by the U.S. Center for Disease Control as one of the greatest public health achievements of the twentieth century be the underlying cause of the modern acne epidemic? You might think dentists are the main characters in that plot, but they only played a supporting role. The question is, who were they supporting? And who was supporting them?

---

[38] *Dr. Strangelove* is a 1964 film that old people point to as evidence that people who disagree with them about fluoride are conspiracy theorists. It might be peer-reviewed but I'm not sure because it seems anecdotal and pro-fluoridationists supposedly aren't into that sort of thing. You can view the scene in question at ProjectFree.Me/Strangelove.

2

F—The Invisible Element Behind the Modern Acne Epidemic

"It started as an observation, that soon took the shape of an idea. It ended, five decades later, as a scientific revolution that shot dentistry into the forefront of preventive medicine. This is the story of how dental science discovered—and ultimately proved to the world—that fluoride, a mineral found in rocks and soil, prevents tooth decay. Although dental caries remains a public health worry, it is no longer the unbridled problem it once was, thanks to fluoride."

—from "The Story of Fluoridation"
National Institute of Dental and Craniofacial Research

A Young Prince in a Shining Castle

THE FULL STORY OF FLUORIDATION CANNOT BE CONTAINED IN A BOOK, let alone a single chapter, but even in the official version—such as the one currently told on the website of the National Institute of Dental and Craniofacial Research (NIDCR)—it is not difficult to see the heart of a deeper story beating just beneath the surface.

According to the official narrative, the story of fluoridation begins with a young dentist who literally rides west and rescues local children from unsightly smiles. I will summarize this version of the story using much of their same wording, or you can read the full account directly on the NIDCR website.[1] See if you can spy any hidden story lines, including the big hairy gorilla who struts across the stage halfway through.

*****

Frederick McCay was a young dental school graduate who left Pennsylvania to open a dental practice in Colorado Springs. When McCay arrived in Colorado, he was astounded to find scores of local citizens with grotesque brown stains on their teeth. He searched in vain for information on the bizarre disorder, but there was a lack of interest among most area dentists. Local residents blamed the problem on any number of strange factors. McCay took up the gauntlet and researched the disorder himself, discovering that teeth afflicted with the brown stain were surprisingly and inexplicably resistant to decay.

McCay didn't know what was causing the brown stain, but that changed when he was contacted by H.V. Churchill, the chief chemist at the Aluminum Company of America (Alcoa). Churchill, who had spent the past few years refuting claims that aluminum was poisonous, conducted a special analysis of the water in Bauxite, a company town owned by Alcoa. (The name of the city was derived from its large reserve of bauxite, a natural material used in the manufacturing of aluminum.) The chemist's analysis identified fluoride as the culprit for the brown stains on children's teeth and he kindly offered "that we may cooperate in an attempt to discover what part 'fluorine' might play in the matter."

Here is where Dr. H. Trendley Dean, head of the Dental Hygiene Unit at the National Institute of Health, enters the stage. Government research on fluoride and its effect on tooth enamel begins in earnest. The architect of these first fluoride studies, Dean makes the critical discovery that fluoride levels up to 1.0 ppm in drinking water do not cause enamel fluorosis in most people. He recalls from McCay's studies that mottled tooth enamel is

---

[1] "The Story of Fluoridation," National Institute of Dental and Craniofacial Research website (available at www.nidcr.nih.gov/oralhealth/Topics/Fluoride/ TheStoryofFluoridation.htm as of May 2016).

unusually resistant to decay and he wonders whether adding fluoride to drinking water would help fight cavities. This hypothesis, Dean tells his colleagues, would need to be tested. Dean got his wish in 1945 when Grand Rapids, Michigan became the first city in the world to fluoridate its drinking water.

The Grand Rapids water fluoridation study was originally sponsored by the U.S. Surgeon General, but was taken over by the National Institute of Dental Research shortly after its inception in 1948, with Dean as the new Institute's director. The results of Dean's 15-year study in Grand Rapids were astounding. Cavities dropped by more than 60 percent after fluoride was added, leading to water fluoridation projects throughout the country that currently benefit over 200 million Americans. Dean's finding was a remarkable feat of science—an achievement ranking with the other great preventative health measures of our century.

*****

A Hollywood fraternity of pre-teen dental groupies could not have imagined a better plot. There's a young altruistic dentist hero. Confused townspeople. Vulnerable children. There's a big mystery, then it's solved. And in the end, a wise government dentist brings health and happiness to millions of people around the globe, establishing American dentistry at the forefront of preventive medicine. If you look closely, however, you'll see clues even the NIDCR story does not hide. The deeper story of fluoridation is not about rescuing people from cavities—it is about *pollution*.

Reading the story above with a skeptical twenty-first century eye, one might be suspicious of the presence of the Alcoa chemist whose bit part was the discovery that fluoride was responsible for the browning of children's teeth. Why was Alcoa studying fluoride, and why was their chief chemist so eager to cooperate with dentists?

One of the most common elements in the earth's crust, fluoride is also the most reactive. Because of its high reactivity, fluoride is not found on its own in nature but is bound with common metals and minerals such as bauxite and phosphate. In addition, fluoride has the prized ability of lowering the melting point of metals, making it a bedrock of key manufacturing processes. This explains why fluoride is a byproduct of so many industries, from aluminum plants and phosphate processors, to steel mills, coal burning operations, and brick and tile manufacturers.

According to the U.S. Department of Agriculture, "Airborne fluorides have caused more worldwide damage to domestic animals than any other air pollutant."[2] Leonard Weinstein, a Cornell professor and international authority on the effect of fluorides in plants, states, "Certainly, there has been more litigation on alleged damage to agriculture by fluoride than all other pollutants combined."[3] Successful lawsuits over fluoride emissions were already a reality in Europe in the late 1800s and industry leaders in the United States correctly predicted they were vulnerable to similar litigation. When dentists started investigating fluoride, corporations were all too willing to work closely with them to keep an eye on the science and help direct their research.

In 1913, Alcoa leaders took this strategy a step further when they created the Mellon Institute of Industrial Research at the University of Pittsburgh. Alcoa-funded researchers at the Mellon Institute were the first to make a public proposal to add fluoride to the water supply.[4] Similarly, the Kettering Laboratory of Applied Physiology at the University of Cincinnati was established in 1930 by other corporations with a self interest in proving the safety of fluoride,

---

[2] "Air Pollutants Affecting the Performance of Domestic Animals," Agricultural Handbook No. 380, U.S. Department of Agriculture, revised 1972, p. 109 (as cited at http://fluoridealert.org/articles/environment-73/).

[3] Weinstein, L.H. "Effects of Fluorides on Plants and Plant Communities: An Overview." 1983, pp. 53-59. In: Shupe, J.L.; Peterson, H.B.; Leone, N.C., (Eds). "Fluorides: Effects on Vegetation, Animals, and Humans." Salt Lake City, UT: Paragon Press, 1983.

[4] For a detailed account of industry's role in fluoridation, see Bryson, Christopher. *The Fluoride Deception.* New York: Seven Stories Press, 2011.

including DuPont and General Motors. By 1931, the majority of the Kettering Laboratory's research focused on fluoride. Researchers from Kettering spent their careers refuting studies that revealed the dangers of fluoride exposure. When their own studies indicated fluoride has severe health consequences, the results were never published and were literally hidden in the basement.[5]

What about the 15-year experiment in Grand Rapids that proved fluoridation safe and effective?[6] The flaws are difficult to hide even from our little layman brains. To give just one obvious example, the study was designed to have a control city so researchers could compare the longterm effects of fluoridation in Grand Rapids with the non-fluoridated city of Muskegon, Michigan. But only five years into the 15-year study, fluoride was added to the public water supply in Muskegon, too. This did not hinder the researchers, though, and they confidently concluded that fluoride caused the drop in dental decay.

The Grand Rapids study is littered with these types of blatant inadequacies. Dr. Hubert Arnold, a statistician from the University of California at Davis, used the early fluoridation trials to demonstrate poor statistical analysis to his students. According to Arnold, the studies "are especially rich in fallacies, improper design, invalid use of statistical methods, omissions of contrary data, and just plain

---

[5] For example, when a metal company lost a lawsuit in 1957 involving fluoride's effect on soft tissue, Kettering researchers were instructed to find evidence to refute future claims. Instead, their 1958 study involving 42 beagle dogs showed fluoride, when inhaled, quickly enters the bloodstream and causes damage to lungs and lymph nodes. Industry lawyers were sent copies of the study but it was hidden from the public until investigative journalist Christopher Bryson combed through the basement archives of the old Kettering Laboratory at the University of Cincinnati decades later.

[6] Dean, H.T. et al. "Studies on mass control of dental caries through fluoridation of the public water supply." Public Health Rep. 1950 Oct 27;65(43):1403-8.

Arnold, F.A. Jr.; Dean, H.T.; Knutson, J.W. "Effect of fluoridated public water supplies on dental caries prevalence." Public Health Rep. 1953 Feb;68(2):141-8.

Arnold, F.A. Jr.; Dean, H.T.; Knutson, J.W. "Effect of fluoridated public water supplies on dental caries prevalence." Public Health Rep. 1956 Jul;71(7):652-8.

muddleheadedness and hebetude."[7]

Without a control city, researchers measuring the rate of dental decay in fluoridated Grand Rapids did not see that the rate of dental decay decreased in non-fluoridated cities as well. Statistical analysis of data from the World Health Organization clearly shows the decline in tooth decay occurred equally in non-fluoridated cities throughout the western world as nutrition improved following the Depression Era.[8]

In June 2015, the Cochrane Group, a U.K.-based organization described in *Newsweek* as "the gold standard of scientific rigor in assessing effectiveness of public health policies,"[9] reviewed every official study they could locate on fluoridation and found that in 97 percent, the risk of bias was high.[10] The Cochrane review concluded there is very little evidence on the effectiveness of water fluoridation for the prevention of dental decay.

Far from "proving to the world" the benefits of fluoridation, as the NIDCR narrative states, most developed countries do not consume artificially fluoridated water, including approximately 97 percent of Western Europe.[11] When Sweden's nobel-prize winning scientist, Dr. Arvid Carlsson, investigated the proposal of water fluoridation for his country, he soon became an outspoken critic of the practice.[12]

---

[7] Letter from Hubert A. Arnold, PhD, University of California (Davis) to Dr. Ernest Newbrun, Medical Sciences Bldg, 653, San Francisco, CA, May 28, 1980 (as cited in *The Case Against Fluoride* by Paul Connett et al.).

[8] "Tooth Decay in Fluoridated versus Non-Fluoridated Countries" available at http://fluoridealert.org/issues/caries/who-data/.

[9] Main, Douglas. "Fluoridation May Not Prevent Cavities, Scientific Review Shows," *Newsweek*, June 29, 2015.

[10] Iheozor-Ejiofor Z, Worthington HV, Walsh T, O'Malley L, Clarkson JE, Macey R, Alam R, Tugwell P, Welch V, Glenny A. "Water fluoridation for the prevention of dental caries." Cochrane Database of Systematic Reviews 2015, Issue 6.

[11] For more information, see "Statements from European Health, Water, and Environment Authorities on Water Fluoridation" at www.fluoridealert.org/content/europe-statements/. Be sure to click the red "Source" link next to each country to view the official response directly from the relevant authority.

[12] "Water Fluoridation Obsolete According to Nobel Prize Scientist." Transcript of interview available at www.fluoridealert.org/content/carlsson-interview/.

"Fluoridation is against all principles of modern pharmacology," Carlsson concluded. "Those nations that are using it should feel ashamed of themselves. It's against science." Even without fluoridation, Sweden experienced the same decline in tooth decay as was observed in heavily fluoridated countries like the United States.[13]

Industry did not rely solely on biased and naive researchers to advance their interests in fluoride—there were lawyers involved, as well. Following a spike in industrial fluoride pollution during World War II, the threat of litigation was overwhelming. "Soon we had claims and lawsuits around aluminum smelters from coast to coast," explained Alcoa's leading fluoride litigator, Frank Seamans.[14]

Seamans responded to the crisis by forming a self-described "Fluorine Lawyers Committee" with fluoride litigators collaborating from U.S. Steel, Monsanto Chemical, the Tennessee River Valley Authority, and several other large corporations vulnerable to fluoride pollution lawsuits. The Fluorine Lawyers Committee met regularly to strategize ways to defuse "the fluoride problem" and they played a strong role in directing fluoride research.[15]

The full effect of industry interest on public fluoridation policy in the United States is impossible to quantify. The corporations most affected by fluoride pollution were the most powerful companies in the world, and vital partners with U.S. military and government officials throughout the world wars. When the U.S. Public Health Service prematurely endorsed public water fluoridation in 1950—ten

---

[13] Connect, Michael. "Tooth Decay Trends in Fluoridated Vs. Unfluoridated Countries," Fluoride Action Network, July 2012 (available at www.fluoridealert.org/studies/caries01/).

[14] F. L. Seamans, "Historical, Economic and Legal aspects of Fluoride," in Shupe et al., eds., *Fluorides*, p. 5 (as cited in *The Fluoride Deception* by Christopher Bryson).

[15] The influence of industry lawyers on fluoride research was blatant. One internal document from Seamans to other members of the Fluorine Lawyers Committee labeled "research re human beings" includes an attachment Seamans sent to medical directors at Kettering "in which an attempt is made to more specifically advise just what the lawyers group wishes them to do." Frank Seamans to Robert Kehoe, April 16, 1957, File 17, Box 42, Kettering Files (as cited in *The Fluoride Deception* by Christopher Bryson).

years *before* the conclusion of Dean's fluoridation trial in Grand Rapids —perhaps it should not have come as a surprise. The decision was made under the leadership of Oscar R. Ewing who was designated as head of the Federal Security Agency over the Public Health Service in 1947. Ewing was a longtime Alcoa lawyer and performed legal work for Alcoa in Washington until 1945.[16]

*****

In Fluoride We Trust

For those who are aware of the dirty history of public water fluoridation, it can be hard to believe the practice is still championed today. If the supporting science is overwhelmingly flawed, why does the practice persist? Biased dentists and callous lawyers could not accomplish such an impressive feat on their own. For that, industry had to bring in the sorcerers.

What the official story of fluoride lacks in sophistication and scientific rigor, it makes up for in marketing magic. In his book *Primal Branding: Create Zealots for Your Brand, Your Company, and Your Future*, Forbes branding expert Patrick Hanlon explains that "brands are belief systems." He identifies seven primal branding elements that inspire fans to rabid addiction. Hanlon refers to these seven factors as primal code. They are the creation story, the leader, the creed, rituals, icons, sacred words, and pagans. When the seven elements of the primal code are firmly in place, a brand resonates deep in the public psyche creating "a belief system and products and services that people can believe in." This is how successful brands become a meaningful part of our culture.

---

[16] Oscar Ewing discussed his work for Alcoa in an interview for the Harry S. Truman Museum. J.R., "Oral History Interview with Oscar R. Ewing," Chapel Hill, NC, April 29, 1969. Available at www.trumanlibrary.org/oralhist/ewing1.htm#86.

Hanlon describes a brand as any product, service, organization, social cause, religion, movement, or other entity searching for popular appeal. In this sense, fluoridation is a brand, and it expertly incorporates every element of the primal branding message. By dissecting the official story of fluoridation from a branding perspective, we see why it has proven resistant to change in the face of sound contradictory science. It is because fluoridation is not a science. It is a religion.

*****

Primal Branding Element #1: The Creation Story

Hanlon describes the creation story as "the foundation of trust" for a new belief system, fulfilling an innate desire to know how we came to be. It often involves a mythic quest or an against-all-odds pursuit, and it is the crucial first step that provides answers to why people should care about you, or your product or service. The NIDCR makes clear their story of fluoridation is also the story of the establishment of the National Institute of Dental Research (the predecessor to the NIDCR) which was founded during the early years of the Grand Rapids experiment. Fluoridation was not just a great discovery dentists claim to have made—it is the creation story for the entire U.S. dental system.

Primal Branding Element #2: The Leader

"All successful belief systems have a person who is the catalyst, the risk taker, the visionary," Hanlon writes. In the story of fluoridation, the leading figure is H. Trendley Dean. Dean was the first director of the National Institute of Dental Research, meaning that in addition to being "the father of fluoridation," he is also the father of government institutionalized dentistry in the United States. Dean was selected for this position specifically because of his work with fluoridation. To question fluoridation is to undermine modern dentistry's founding father.

Primal Branding Element #3: The Creed

The creed is the singular notion a brand wants people to believe. It is based on a set of core principles that define a company's mission and explains who they are and why they exist. With the story of fluoridation, dentists brand themselves as heroes rescuing a helpless population from dental decay. To underline this notion, they repeat mantras such as "fluoride is safe and effective" and "fluoridation is one of the greatest public health achievements of the twentieth century" with blind faith in the institutionalized belief system from which such claims originated.

Primal Branding Element #4: Sacred Words

"All belief systems come with a set of specialized words that must be learned before people can belong," Hanlon states. The medical community is infamous for such jargon. For example, while non-dentists speak of cavities and tooth decay, dentists use the term "dental caries." Caries is simply the Latin word for "rottenness," but peer-reviewed publications on the rate of "dental rottenness" would not sound quite as professional. Those who buy into a brand use sacred words as protection for the group's ideals, since they assume members of the group are the only ones who can speak the language. For example, early in the fluoridation effort, the American Dental Association (ADA) advised dentists that fluoridation "should not be submitted to the voters, who cannot possibly sift through and comprehend the scientific evidence."[17]

Primal Branding Element #5: Rituals

Rituals are repeated interactions consumers have with a brand. They are touch points that solidify the brand in the lives of its supporters and highlight the brand's meaning and relevance. The incorporation of both daily and intermittent rituals anchor the fluoride brand firmly in American culture. Adding fluoride to toothpaste brought the twice-daily ritual of fluoride into our homes. We are also chided to visit the dentist twice per year to soak our teeth in fluoride. Marketers now recognize that internal branding is also fundamental to a brand's success. For dentists,

---

[17] Bryson, *The Fluoride Deception.*

the use of fluoride trays is a daily ritual they perform on their patients while an example of an annual ritual is the celebration of the birth of fluoridation. (As I write this paragraph on September 11, 2015, dentists are attending the "70th Anniversary Fluoridation Celebration and Symposium" in Chicago, IL.)

Primal Branding Element #6: Icons

Hanlon describes icons as "quick concentrations of meaning that cause your brand identity and brand values to spontaneously resonate." Often icons are visual, but they can be any sensory trigger that summons the basic substance of the brand. The fluoride logo currently displayed on the homepage for the American Dental Association is a perfect example. Next to a tagline that reads "Fluoride to the rescue!" is a sparkly white tooth with a T superhero emblem on its chest (notice they didn't use an F). Flexing its muscular arms, the tooth is surrounded by little bubbles of sodium fluoride indicated by the periodic symbols F and Na. The entire logo, of course, is red, white, and blue. The icons for fluoridation are not always so cartoonish. A tube of toothpaste is an iconic symbol of fluoride's pervasiveness in American culture. The dentist's waiting room with its requisite magazines, even the dentist's chair—these are icons that evoke the notion of dental authority and reinforce the brand's message of dentist as hero.

Primal Branding Element #7: Pagans and Non-Believers

Pagans are the final element in the primal marketing code. "Defining your pagans is important in defining who you are," Hanlon writes. Recent examples are 7Up declaring itself "the uncola" and Taco Bell urging its audience to "think outside the bun." Believers serve both as brand evangelist and defender. When the brand is threatened, they protect it as if they are the ones under attack. Believers who express doubt are excommunicated and exiled to the opposing camp. This explains why pro-fluoridationists fixate on the caricature of anti-fluoride conspiracy theorists depicted in *Dr. Strangelove*, and why decades of contradictory research barely made a dent in fluoride's superhero status. By pushing against a fanatical belief system, opponents unwittingly make it stronger.

*****

When fluoridation is viewed as a belief system, not a science, it becomes apparent why the practice continues today. Successful brands "fulfill genuine pieces of the human psyche," Hanlon writes. "Believing is belonging."

Questioning the fluoride brand inherently translates as an attack on the entire U.S. dental culture. Its creation story, leader, creed, sacred words, rituals, icons, and pagans are all wrapped up in the story of fluoridation. H. Trendley Dean could not have been a shoddy researcher; he was the founding father. Fluoridation could not have been a ploy by fluoride polluters; it is the NIDCR's reason for existence. How can fluoride be bad for your health if the majority of the U.S. population drinks eight glasses a day?

Sigmund Freud himself could not have conceived of a more brilliant psychological strategy to inculcate American minds with the notion that it is a good idea to put toxic waste from aluminum plants directly into the water supply—but his nephew could.

It is not a coincidence that one of the most controversial public health practices of the twenty-first century is also one of the most successful brands in modern history. All seven pieces of the primal marketing code did not fall into place by happenstance. It was by design. The designer was Edward Bernays who earned his title as the "Father of Public Relations" by combining insights from the burgeoning field of crowd psychology with ideas from psychoanalysis as developed by his uncle, Sigmund Freud.

Bernay's most famous campaign involved staging a group of women suffragists to march in the Easter parade in New York City holding lit cigarettes in the air as "torches of freedom." Women were previously banned from smoking in public outside of designated areas, but by turning smoking into a women's suffragist issue, the publicity from Bernays' campaign helped tobacco companies break a social taboo that was impeding their entry into a mainstream market.

Bernays' work on fluoridation is less well known but even more ingenious. Again, his efforts in New York City provide a brilliant example of his campaign tactics. "If New York City accepts an idea, the other states will accept the idea too," he told journalist Christopher Bryson, author of *The Fluoride Deception,* in a 1993 interview. The fluoridation debate raged in New York in the early 1960s and was described by the *New York Times* as "one of the most contentious issues of the Cold War."[18] The anti-fluoridation movement had successfully stalled fluoridation for several years and was led by leading physicians such as Simon Beisler, former president of the American Urological Association, and Fred Squier Dunn, chief of the Dental Department at the renowned Lenox Hill Hospital in Manhattan.

In a 1960 letter written to the New York Health Commissioner, Bernays describes the public relations strategy he helped implement for fluoridation.[19] In the letter, he counsels the Health Commissioner to write to television executives at NBC and CBS and tell them debating fluoridation "is like presenting two sides for anti-Catholicism or anti-Semitism and therefore not in the public interest." He warns her not to ask them to act in a specific way, but to generally plant the idea in their minds that fluoridation should not be debated. "This might lead to a revision of the whole policy of what shall and shall not be considered controversial," Bernays predicts.

The campaign included sending government letters to influential newspaper editors and even publishers of dictionaries and encyclopedias. The letters were not to argue for fluoridation or address concerns of critics; their intent was to leverage government influence to dominate the fluoridation narrative and marginalize opposition. In this way, pro-fluoridationists manipulated the human tendency to defer to authority sources, such as doctors, dictionaries, and the daily

---

[18] Blumenthal, Ralph. "New York's Fluoridation Fuss, 50 Years Later." *The New York Times,* February 23, 2015.

[19] Bernays to Baumgartner, February 16, 1961, Baumgartner file, ELB papers, Library of Congress (as cited in *The Fluoride Deception* by Christopher Bryson).

news. Bernays referred to this technique as the *engineering of consent* which relies on *third party authorities* to give credence to a brand or product. "You can get practically any idea accepted," Bernays told Bryson. "If doctors are in favor, the public is willing to accept it, because a doctor is an authority to most people, regardless of how much he knows, or doesn't know... By the law of averages, you can usually find an individual in any field who will be willing to accept new ideas."

In his seminal book *Propaganda,* Bernays describes his philosophy behind the engineering of consent further. "Those who manipulate this unseen mechanism of society constitute an invisible government which is the true ruling power of our country," he writes. "It is they who pull the wires which control the public mind."

Bernays spent his retirement in penance supporting anti-smoking campaigns, claiming he would have refused to work with the tobacco industry if he knew of the negative health effects of cigarettes earlier. He seems not to have realized that even while helping to pull the strings, he was part of the public mind that was being controlled.

*****

Patrons and Pagans

Once a belief system is manifest in government institutions, it becomes deeply entrenched in a culture and, like a mastodon in quicksand, nearly impossible to budge. It's not that present-day government officials and dentists are evil beings who knowingly poison the entire population to protect their precious fluoridation scheme. They are regular people who see what they expect to see and feel safe when siding with the majority and the status quo.

The longer a brand is established, the more layered it becomes as complementary entities grow around it and reinforce the belief structure. These patrons can be offshoots of the brand or entirely separate entities that gravitate to the brand because they share a common interest. In the story of fluoridation, we find both types.

One such patron is the dental hygiene industry. Fluoridated toothpaste is a dream product for an entrepreneur. It must be repurchased on a regular and frequent basis, it has a price point that makes it both accessible to the masses and massively profitable, and it is endorsed by third party authorities as an indispensable part of daily life for everyone, everywhere—not just once a day, but two times or more.[20]

Proctor & Gamble (P&G) set out to dominate the fluoride toothpaste market when it launched the Crest brand in the 1950s, originally marketed under the unfortunate name Fluoristan. Renamed as Crest with Fluoristan, the new line was unveiled with an ad campaign featuring Norman Rockwell paintings of gleeful children proudly waving their dental check-up cards. The campaign tagline, "Look, Mom—no cavities!" raised concerns at the time about truth in advertising. At a congressional hearing in 1958, the assistant secretary for the American Dental Association's (ADA) Counsel on Dental Therapeutics claimed the ads were "at best both a gross exaggeration and a misleading distortion."[21]

Just two years later (the same year Bernays started his fluoridation campaign for the New York Health Commissioner), the ADA suddenly changed its mind about Crest and selected it as the first and only toothpaste to receive the ADA seal of approval. Within one year of the announcement, Crest more than doubled its share of the toothpaste market. As an added benefit, future truth in advertising complaints were circumvented simply by referring to the ADA endorsement as proof that Crest fights cavities.

---

[20] For an enlightening account of how marketers hooked the world on foamy mint toothpaste, see *The Power of Habit: Why We Do What We Do in Life and Business* by Charles Duhigg.

[21] McDonough, John and Karen Egolf, eds. *The Advertising Age: Encyclopedia of Advertising.* Chicago: Fitzroy Dearborn Publishers, 2002.

Now that Crest was widely profitable, P&G took over the marketing of fluoride where Bernays' campaign left off. Until the 1980s, P&G spent more money on advertising for Crest than any other brand in its extensive lineup, including Tide laundry detergent, Ivory soap, and Pampers diapers.[22] By the end of the twentieth century, the company was spending upwards of $90 million *per year* on advertising for Crest products, ensuring the official story of fluoride remained deeply instilled in the American psyche.

Financial proceeds from fluoridated products continue to find their way back to government supporters through grants and donations, strategic partnerships, and industry-sponsored non-profit organizations.[23] In 2014, Crest toothpaste alone generated over $380 million in sales.[24]

Other patrons of fluoridation are not as overt. In November 2007, Cristin Kearns, a dental administrator for Kaiser Permanente's Dental Care Program, attended a conference in Seattle intended to educate dentists on the links between diabetes and gum disease. She was confused when the keynote speaker, Dr. Stephen Aldana, insisted "there is no research to support that sugar causes chronic disease." Her experience working in low-income dental clinics in Denver told her otherwise.

Kearns suspected the sugar industry might be manipulating the nutritional advice dental professionals like herself were receiving. A google search for "International Sugar Research Foundation" and

---

[22] *Ibid.*

[23] Such as the Friends of NIDCR, a non-profit organization whose mission is "to educate the public and key decision makers about the importance of investing in the NIDCR." To return the sentiment, at their annual conference in Washington, DC, Friends of NIDCR hosts an industry roundtable whose mission is "to drive awareness amongst the oral health community of the role that industry plays in the success of Public/Private Partnerships (PPPs)." The first roundtable was chaired by Dr. J. Leslie Winston, scientific relations director at Procter and Gamble Company. See "DTA to Sponsor Friends of NIDCR Industry Roundtable 'Public/Private Partnerships.'"

[24] See "Sales of the leading toothpaste brands in the United States in 2014" at Statista.com (available at www.statista.com/statistics/195650/leading-us-toothpaste-brands-in-2007-and-2008-based-on-sales/).

"archives" led her to a neglected trove of firsthand evidence of the subversive role the sugar industry had long been playing in dental research. The University of Illinois librarian who archived the files from a bankrupt sugar company thought they mostly documented the impact of the beet sugar industry on farm labor, but as Kearns soon realized, they documented much more than that.

The cache of internal documents, which Kearns quit her job to study, revealed the sugar industry's shockingly close ties with the National Institute of Dental Research in the 1960s and '70s while it was building the National Caries Program, an initiative implemented under President Nixon in 1971 with the goal of ending dental decay in a decade.

In March 2015, Kearns, now a postdoctoral fellow at the University of California San Francisco (UCSF), published a paper with her findings in the peer-reviewed journal *PLoS Medicine*.[25] Along with her two co-authors, Kearns revealed the NIDR steering committee tasked with prioritizing research initiatives for dental decay was composed almost entirely of personnel from the International Sugar Research Foundation's (ISRF) Scientific Advisory Board whose stated purpose was "to discover effective means of controlling tooth decay by methods *other* than restricting carbohydrate intake" (emphasis added). The sugar industry needed dentists to focus on a way to strengthen teeth so they would be distracted from identifying the true cause of dental decay—which is not a lack of fluoride, but an excess of sugar.

As with the fluoride polluters decades before, the sugar industry encouraged fluoride as a dental treatment to hide evidence of its own vulnerability. The internal documents reveal industry scientists were well aware of sugar's leading role in dental decay as early as 1950, and they promoted programs on enzymes, dental vaccines, and fluoride in an effort to deflect attention from sugar as the culprit.

---

[25] Kearns, Cristin E., Glantz, Stanton A., and Laura A. Schmidt. "Sugar Industry Influence on the Scientific Agenda of the National Institute of Dental Research's 1971 National Caries Program: A Historical Analysis of Internal Documents," *PLoS Medicine*, March 2015.

When the National Caries Program submitted their omnibus request for contracts in 1971, which set the precedent for the direction dental research would take for the years ahead, the authors of the request copied verbatim or closely paraphrased 78 percent of a report the sugar industry submitted to the NIDR two years earlier.[26]

While the patrons of fluoridation are behemoth billion-dollar juggernauts, the pagans are quite the opposite: individuals who, through circumstance, became aware of the inaccuracies, inadequacies, and injustices of the fluoridation story and decided to speak up about it. They have limited financial backing, political influence, or media access and thus are easily dismissed, crucified, or ignored altogether. Much of their efforts have been bulldozed by the fluoride faithful who cling to the creed that "fluoridation is safe and effective" and block out all evidence to the contrary. Pro-fluoridationists want to believe (and want you to believe) that qualified critics of fluoridation do not exist, but the following vignettes offer a glimpse of some of the protagonists on the other side of the fluoridation story through the years.

*****

Kaj Roholm: Cryolite mines in Denmark made the country an early testbed for fluoride pollution. Roholm, the Deputy Health Commissioner of Copenhagen, authored the 1937 tome *Fluoride Intoxication*, a monumental study of the toxic effects of fluoride, including a 40-page bibliography with 893 references to scientific articles. Roholm noted the amount of fluoride recommended in the United States to prevent tooth decay was close to the toxic limit and warned, "The particular danger in the therapeutic use of fluorine compounds is the development of a chronic intoxication." Recognized as the world's leading expert on fluoride toxicity, Roholm was unable to defend his work from the inevitable harsh criticism it received in the U.S. during the early fluoridation era due to his untimely death from cancer in 1948.

---

[26] *Ibid.*

George Waldbott: After graduating from medical school in Germany, Waldbott accepted a residency in Michigan where he embarked on a pioneering career in the study and treatment of allergic diseases. Beginning in the 1950s, he published numerous research papers that indicated a significant portion of the population is hyper-sensitive to fluoride. He spent the rest of his life advocating against public water fluoridation, founding the International Society for Fluoride Research and its quarterly journal, *Fluoride*. Described as an "eminent" allergist even by his critics,[27] official studies were never attempted to refute his findings.

Phyllis Mullenix: After receiving her doctorate in pharmacology, Mullenix worked at Johns Hopkins School of Public Health and then Harvard Medical School until she was selected to establish the toxicology department at the Forsyth Dental Center in Boston in 1983, the first toxicology department in any dental institution in the world. After her supervisor encouraged her to study fluoride, she was surprised when the science indicated fluoride is a neurotoxin. She was even more surprised when health officials ignored her research and cut off her funding. She was then fired from her position at Forsyth.[28]

John Colquhoun: An ardent fluoridation advocate, Colquhoun was chairman of New Zealand's "Fluoridation Promotion Committee" when research on fluoride started to raise questions in his mind about its safety and effectiveness. He reversed his stance on fluoride in the early 1980s, a move that cost him his prestigious position as the Principal Dental Officer of Aukland, the country's largest city. In 1991, Colquhoun became the editor of *Fluoride* and a board member of the International Society of Fluoride Research. He outlined his reasons for opposing fluoridation in a 1997 article published in *Perspectives in Biology and Medicine* by Johns Hopkins University Press.[29]

---

[27] Prival, MJ. "Fluorides and human health." Center for Science in the Public Interest, Washington D.C.,1972, pp. 23-25.

[28] Connett, Paul. "Fluoride & the Brain: An Interview with Dr. Phyllis Mullenix," October 18, 1997 (available at www.fluoridealert.org/content/mullenix-interview/).

[29] Colquhoun, John. "Why I Changed My Mind About Water Fluoridation." *Perspectives in Biology and Medicine*, 41, 1, Autumn 1997.

William Marcus: A leading toxicologist at the EPA's Office of Drinking Water, Marcus was fired in 1992 after raising health concerns about fluoride. He filed a lawsuit under the Whistleblower Protection Act and after a fierce two-year court battle prevailed on every count. He was reinstated to his job at the EPA but continued to experience harassment, later filing and winning a second hearing over his hostile work environment. Court evidence revealed collusion between EPA managers and numerous chemical companies.[30] Marcus' health concerns over fluoride were never addressed in EPA policy.

Hardy Limeback: Former president of the Canadian Association for Dental Research, Limeback headed the Department of Preventive Dentistry at the University of Toronto. After publishing numerous papers on the benefits of fluoridation and serving as a consultant on fluoride to the Canadian Dental Association, Limeback, who has a doctorate in collagen biochemistry, changed his position on fluoridation in the 1990s after examining the effect of ingested fluorides on bone development.[31] He was subsequently passed over by Canadian health officials from participating in future fluoridation reviews.

William Hirzy: A senior scientist at EPA's Office of Pollution Prevention and Toxics, Hirzy was also President of the EPA Headquarters Union. His attention turned to fluoride in 1985 when EPA was revising its drinking water standard for fluoride. An employee complained to the Union that he was being coerced to write an assessment he did not support. For the rest of his career, Hirzy represented 1,500 EPA professionals in opposing fluoridation. He even testified before the U.S. Senate on behalf of the Union in June 2000 regarding the Union's rejection of public water fluoridation.[32]

---

[30] For more information, see the summary of Dr. Marcus' case at the website of Kohn, Kohn, and Colapinto, LLP available at www.kkc.com, or see an interview with Dr. Marcus available at http://fluoridealert.org/content/marcus-interview/.

[31] The letter Limeback wrote to explain the reasons for his change in stance include references to 143 scientific articles. See, Limeback, Hardy. "Why I Am Now Officially Opposed to Adding Fluoride To Drinking Water." Apr 2000 (available at www.fluoridealert.org/articles/limeback/.)

[32] See Hirzy, J. William. "Why EPA's Headquarters Professionals' Union Opposes Fluoridation," 2000 (available at www.fluoridealert.org/articles/epa-union/). View video of Hirzy's senate testimony at ProjectFree.Me/Hirzy.

Paul Connett: With degrees from Cambridge and Dartmouth, Connett was a professor of chemistry and toxicology for 23 years at St. Lawrence University before retiring to found the Fluoride Action Network (FAN) in May 2000, a non-profit organization dedicated to raising awareness of the health effects of fluoride exposure. Connett and the FAN team gather the latest news and research on fluoride, provide input to policy makers, and support local anti-fluoridation campaigners. (The research gathered on FAN's extensive website, fluoridealert.org, was invaluable in healing my acne.)

*****

These are just a few of the perfectly credentialed scientists whose voices have been marginalized by fluoridation proponents. I am tempted to continue with other examples because their stories are important, but they always have the same plot. Non-believers suggest fluoridation has negative health effects and call for research and caution, while dentists point to a lack of evidence and cite the creed —"more than [x] years of scientific research has consistently shown that an optimal level of fluoride in community water is safe and effective."[33]

If this is the first time you are learning about the underground story of fluoridation, you might be feeling disheartened, angry, powerless, or in a state of disbelief. With fluoridation so deeply entrenched in American culture, how can individuals like you and me ever hope to change it?

Not to worry. There is a plan.[34] In the meantime, to heal your acne, you do not need to change anything that is not already well within your reach to change. You just need to turn the page.

---

[33] This phrase was taken directly from the CDC webpage on fluoridation on September 19, 2015 (available at www.ada.org/en/public-programs/advocating-for-the-public/fluoride-and-fluoridation).

[34] See Afterword: Ending Acne. Also, **ProjectFree.Me/STOP**.

3

RETHINKING THE CAUSE OF YOUR ACNE

LET'S RECAP. ESKIMOS START EXPERIENCING ACNE when they move to town. Dermatologists develop a drug addiction. Native Kitavans never get acne. The Ache don't either. Paleo godfather ALMOST cures acne. Dentists create a fluoride cult. Avoiding fluoride cures my acne. That brings us to the current point in our story. Here is where your part comes in.

*****

Tales from Gotham City

After my fluoride epiphany in 2008, I tested my fluoride hypothesis on my own skin so many times the results were undeniable, even for family members who originally thought I was crazy when I told them tap water makes my skin break out (be forewarned, family members tend to do that). It took a few years for me to figure out how to reduce my exposure enough to heal my chronic acne for good, but by 2010 my breakouts were nonexistent.

Along the way, I was writing about my experience on my blog, The Cellulite Investigation, and almost immediately, some of the people who read my posts on acne said they also started noticing breakouts from fluoride. It was strange. I assumed fluoride-induced acne was an obscure condition. I never heard of it before. None of the experts I consulted over the years mentioned it. The scientific literature was sparse. Even Internet didn't seem to know much about it.

In 2011, I posted a free guide on my site explaining the basics of fluoride and acne. Keep in mind, most people who visited the site did so because of their interest in cellulite, not acne. I typically received only a couple hundred visitors per day, and my bounce rate (the amount of people who leave without looking around) was consistently close to 70 percent. That's not good. Even my most popular acne post only received a handful of views per day, if any. However, despite my total lack of blogging skills, I started to receive success stories from other people who cured their cystic acne by avoiding fluoride.

It should have been highly improbable that someone suffering from acne would (1) find my website, (2) read my guide, (3) implement my recommendations, (4) heal their acne, and (5) come back to tell me about it. I did some quick math. If I already heard from this many people with fluoride-induced acne, how many more of us were out there?

Over the next few years, in addition to the testimonials coming in from visitors to my website, I caught glimpses of the gorilla around town more and more. A man on the plane with deep welts down his chin and neck. A young woman at work with heavy makeup trying to hide cysts along her jawline. The gorilla was hanging out all over the online acne forums, too. The experts all pinky swore never ever to read health information on the internet, *especially* the comments and forums. But intelligence analysts and other trained investigators know, sometimes your best source for intel is the man on the street.

Before I am written up by the science hall monitors, I realize each of the comments I am about to show you are anecdotal (not in the pejorative sense). None of the commenters suspect fluoride as the cause of their acne, and even if they did, their suspicions would likely be speculative. And yes, with the gajillions of comments on the internet, you could likely find at least a couple to support the theory that acne is caused by rainbow kryptonite. These are all valid points. I am not trying to *prove* fluoroderma exists by cherry picking anecdotal evidence from the internet. The accounts below are simply a few real-world *illustrations* that I am incorporating into my larger proposition that fluoride-induced acne is not an uncommon condition—and that we will only recognize it once we know to look. My aim with this book is to encourage other people, like you, to start looking. (In the comments that follow, I'm pointing at the gorilla *like this*.)

*****

Belmondo writes at "Acne Anecdotes" on WholeHealthSource:[1] But why oh why do I still get spots?! I'm doing everything right nutritionally. I've been lowcarbing for years (*I'm 30*)… But I still get spots weekly. I eat a high fat, high protein, animal based diet, the few carbs coming from *potatoes* and *rice* mostly. Completely gluten free for two months now, has made no difference. I've started on vitamin D and zinc recently like Cordain suggests in his Acne book. No difference… Also, is there a difference between different places to have spots? I most often have mine in the area *from the corner of mouth down to the jaw*.

> **Stephan Guyenet replies:** wish I had an answer for you. All I can think of is increasing your vitamin A intake (liver, cod liver oil). Anyone else have suggestions?

> **Belmondo replies:** As to vit A, I usually try to eat liver every week, I take cod liver oil in the winter, and use plenty of vitamin A-rich foods such as butter.

> **mess talker replies:** I was getting some *weird rash around my mouth* and it went away when I stopped using Mint *toothpaste*. Years later.

---

[1] Comments posted at "Acne Anecdotes" by Stephen Guyenet at WholeHealthSource. Blogspot.com, Oct 4, 2008 (available at http://wholehealthsource.blogspot.com/2008/10/acne-anecdotes.html).

Belmondo writes at "Reversing Tooth Decay" on WholeHealthSource:[2] (six months later in a different post) Stephan, I'd love to hear your opinion on *fluoride*? Helpful or harmful?

> **Stephan Guyenet replies:** I haven't really formed a strong opinion on fluoride yet, except that it's bizarre that the government is allowed to conduct *involuntary mass medication*... But I don't know if I'm going to go there on the blog because *it's an inflammatory topic*.

Elizabeth writes at "I Gave Up Dairy and All I Got Was the Best Skin of My Life" on XOJane:[3] I recently had a maddening experience with acne. I had the *deep cystic kind around my jawline that began suddenly* when *I turned 23*. I did everything right, I stopped wheat, sugar and dairy and went to a doctor to get my hormones addressed... *Over christmas break* I did everything wrong! alcohol, wheat, sugar, dairy in abundance ... GUESS WHAT!? In time for my 25th birthday my skin cleared to an angelic glow of epic proportions... Sometimes there is no logic whatsoever!!!!

> **Annie replies:** ...you were less stressed—perhaps that's the reason for the improvement?

> **Elizabeth replies:** Perhaps, but I was having anxiety attacks almost daily being with my mom!

---

[2] Comments posted at "Reversing Tooth Decay" by Stephen Guyenet at WholeHealth Source.blogspot.com, Apr 9, 2009 (available at WholeHealthSource.blogspot.com/2009/03/reversing-tooth-decay.html).

[3] Comments posted at "I Gave Up Dairy And All I Got Was The Best Skin Of My Life" by Annie Tomlin at XOJane.com, Jan 31, 2014 (available at www.xojane.com/beauty/i-gave-up-dairy-and-all-i-got-was-the-best-skin-of-my-life).

> **lostYouTh06 writes at "chlorine and acne... what i've experienced" on HealthBoards:[4]** over the past *two years* i have had pretty *persistent acne* on my face. i wash my face two times a day, am on a pretty healthy-conscious diet, and *drink a lot of water*... but that still never seems to really help. ...but to get to the point, it was very hot this past summer. i had not gone swimming all year. my family took a *vacation* to texas and we spent a lot of time at a water park near our hotel. i hadn't gone swimming all summer and i noticed after *two days* at the water park my face had cleared up. i hadn't even been washing it on the vacation except for taking a shower every night. it was amazing, it had to be *something in the water*.

> **blackie writes at "Acne Paleo-Inuit-Ache-Masai-Kitava Diet" on Paleohacks:[5]** My *cystic acne* erupted badly the last time when i eat *raisins* and apple together... darn it! i loved *raisins* so much.

*****

Poor blackie. If only he knew that selecting truly *organic* raisins would solve his star-crossed love affair with shriveled grapes. In California, where virtually all the raisins in the United States originate, grape vines are intentionally coated with fluoride because it kills the insects that destroy grape crops. It is a pesticide known as cryolite. More on that later.

Anecdotal has become a curse word in the modern medical world, but the experiences of individuals, like you and me and those

---

[4] Comments posted at "chlorine and acne... what i've experienced" by lostYouTh06 at HealthBoards.com, Jan 23, 2005 (available at www.healthboards.com/boards/acne/245690-chlorine-acne-what-ive-experienced.html).

[5] Comment posted at "ACNE Paleo-Inuit-Ache-Masai-Kitava Diet" by blackie at PaleoHacks.com, Feb 20, 2011 (available at www.paleohacks.com/paleo/acne-paleo-inuit-ache-masai-kitava-diet-3201).

described above, have their place in scientific inquiry. The Cambridge dictionary defines anecdotal information as "not based on facts or careful study." What?! According to Merriam-Webster, it means "based on or consisting of reports or observations of usually unscientific observers." But the etymology of the word suggests something different.

The word "anecdotal" goes back to the ancient Greek idea of *anekdota*, from *an-*, "not," and *ekdota*, "published." The meaning of anecdotal started to change when Procopius, the last major historian of the ancient world, used it as the title of his scandalous account of the venal and salacious private lives of Roman emperor Justinian and his wife, Theodora. (See what Procopius did there? He took a word that meant *unpublished* and he published it. That Procopius!) His book, based on court gossip, gave the word *anecdotal* a sense of "revelation of secrets" which then degraded in English into "brief, amusing stories" and finally "dubious support of a generalized claim," as anecdotal evidence is currently described on Wikipedia.

But an alternative definition in Merriam-Webster describes anecdotal as "of, relating to, or being the depiction of a scene suggesting a story." With this definition, we see more clearly the value anecdotal evidence can offer to those who are astute and humble enough to listen.

In an article published in the *Lancet,* entitled "Value of Anecdotes," Rodger Charlton points out, "Publication in a scientific peer-viewed medical journal is unlikely to follow anecdotal observation. And yet in the *Lancet* of 1923 such observations were commonplace and at a time when major medical discoveries were being made."[6] Anecdotes are not anathema to scientific progress. They are the starting point. They are scenes that suggest a story. At their heart, anecdotes are single observations in the physical world—and that is where science must always begin.

---

[6] Charlton, Rodger. "Value of Anecdotes." *The Lancet,* Vol.355, No. 9212, Apr 15, 2000, p. 1372.

Returning to the anecdotal evidence I know best—my own—there is much information that can be mined from my experience with acne that you can use as a starting point to ascertain if fluoride is the source of your acne as well. First, let's talk demographics. I am a thirty-something adult and I am female. There is a common misperception that acne is a rite of passage for teenagers. This might have been the case a generation ago when fluoride was not as pervasive and older generations did not grow up with fluoridated teeth and bones. This is not the reality today.

Dermatologists and my hairdresser have both noticed the rise in adult acne, especially with women.[7] In a 2012 study published in the *Journal of Women's Health*, researchers from Harvard Medical School recruited 2,895 females aged 10 to 70 from the general population and found that 55 percent had some form of acne, including 45 percent of women aged 21 to 30, 26 percent aged 31 to 40, and 12 percent aged 41 to 50.[8]

Acne can continue from adolescence or it can start in later years, a condition dermatologists refer to as late-onset acne. Dermatologists do not have an explanation for the observed increase in late-onset acne or for the rise in adult acne in general. However, this phenomenon is consistent with the fluoride theory of acne since it has long been recognized that fluoride accumulates in bone over time.[9]

---

[7] Dreno, B., "Treatment of adult female acne: a new challenge," *Journal of the European Academy of Dermatology and Venereology,* Vol. 29, Issue S5, Jun 2015, pp. 14–19.

[8] Perkins, Alexis C. et al. "Acne Vulgaris in Women: Prevalence Across the Life Span." *Journal of Women's Health,* Vol. 21(2), Feb 2012, pp. 223-23.

[9] In parts of the world such as India and China where fluoride occurs naturally in drinking water, skeletal fluorosis is a common and debilitating condition and has been observed in areas where fluoride concentrations are equivalent to the current CDC recommendation for "optimally" fluoridated water. SOURCE: Dai, G. et al. "Distributive regulation of bone substance change in various population sub-groups with different fluoride concentrations in drinking water." *Chinese Journal of Endemiology,* 2004. For more information, see Connett, Michael. "Skeletal Fluorosis in India and China" Fluoride Action Network, May 2012 (available at www.fluoridealert.org/studies/skeletal_fluorosis05/).

The more fluoride we consume, the more the rate of adult acne will increase.

The placement of your acne is another clue. Like Belmondo describes in his comment to Stephan Guyenet, I often developed acne in a line from the corners of my nose and mouth down to the bottom of my chin. Sometimes when dermatologists see this pattern they diagnose it as perioral dermatitis. *Peri-* is from Greek and means around. *Oral*, of course, means pertaining to the mouth. Dermatitis comes from *derma-*, skin, and *-itis*, inflammation. So when a dermatologist says you have perioral dermatitis, it's really just Greek caveman-speak for "around mouth, skin bad, take drug."

Sometimes the lines of my acne breakouts extended from my nose all the way down the front of my neck, onto my chest. In a 2013 article entitled "Adult Female Acne: A New Paradigm," the authors note that in the rising tide of adult acne, "lesions are generally more prominent on the lower chin, jawline and neck."[10] This pattern makes perfect sense since fluoride accumulates in the teeth and jaw, and then we brush, swish, and gargle with it twice a day. When my fluoroderma was at its worst, I also developed lines of acne from my ears down the sides of my neck, and from the base of my skull down the back of my neck. Sometimes I even developed clusters of acne on my forehead, and painful lumps around my ears and inside my earlobes.

A major clue in my self-diagnosis of fluoroderma was the realization that my breakouts were related to travel. Within two days of arriving at a new location, it was clear whether or not the new setting was going to be "one of those places." If your acne is conspicuously affected by travel, or if you notice a sudden onset or clearing of breakouts after moving to a new location, then that is an indicator your acne might be caused by fluoride. Once the idea of fluoroderma entered my mind, I was easily able to look back over my

---

[10] Dreno, B., "Adult Female Acne: A New Paradigm." *Journal of the European Academy of Dermatology and Venereology*, Vol. 27, Issue 9, Sep 2013, pp. 1063–1070.

experience and see if my worst bouts of acne coincided with the cities where I was exposed to a higher level of fluoride. You can research whether or not towns are fluoridated by calling the local water municipality or looking up their annual water quality report online (also known as consumer confidence reports). Public water utilities are required by law to provide this information.

Another clue was my preexisting dental fluorosis. Remember the "grotesque brown stains" on local's teeth in the NIDCR's story of fluoridation? As the story goes, "So severe could these permanent stains be, in fact, sometimes entire teeth were splotched the color of chocolate candy."[11] (Leave it to dentists to come up with this analogy.) The extent of dental fluorosis seen today is rarely so severe, but any dentist will be able to recognize it. My dental fluorosis appears as bright white spots on the face of my teeth and an opaque quality around the edges. During my routine checkups, several dentists have also pointed out pitting and deep crevices, likely caused by the fluoride pills prescribed for me as a child.

Dental fluorosis only develops when fluoride is ingested in early childhood, when teeth are still being formed. When my permanent teeth came in, my parents asked my pediatrician about the discoloration, but he did not know the cause. I also developed chronic nose bleeds at this time, another indicator of fluoride toxicity. A survey released by the CDC in 2010 revealed 41 percent of adolescents aged 12 to 15 have dental fluorosis—that is roughly *twice* the rate they found in the same age group the decade prior.[12] Dental authorities insist the condition is purely cosmetic. But as my favorite pagan dentist, Hardy Limeback, has stated, "It is illogical to assume that tooth enamel is the only tissue affected by low daily doses of fluoride ingestion."[13]

---

[11] "The Story of Fluoridation," NIDCR website.

[12] Beltran, E.D., et al. "Prevalence and Severity of Dental Fluorosis in the United States, 1999-2004." NCHS Data Brief No. 53, Nov 2010.

[13] Limeback, Hardy. "Why I Am Now Officially Opposed to Adding Fluoride To Drinking Water." Apr 2000 (available at www.fluoridealert.org/articles/limeback/.)

None of the indicators above will prove or disprove that your acne is caused by fluoride. Not all adult females have fluoroderma and not everyone with fluoroderma is an adult female. Perhaps the location of my breakouts is specific to my particular history with fluoride and how it accumulated in my bones, teeth, and tissues. Maybe you don't have dental fluorosis, but you were exposed to high amounts of fluoride after your permanent teeth developed. Maybe your travels have not taken you to places where there was a significant difference in the amount of fluoride in the water supply, or maybe you consumed high amounts of fluoride that occurs naturally in some well water or from food sources.

That's the thing with anecdotal evidence. It requires further study to see how the observations drawn from one instance can be applied to others. You will need to figure out that part on your own. But because I *really, really, really* want to help you with it, I will tell you some other indicators of fluoroderma that are wrapped up in a dark secret I've scarcely whispered to a soul. They involve a side of acne that few people talk about, but even the experts have noticed.

PurplGrind writes at "University and Acne?" on Acne.org:[14]
I've been at university for two weeks now and my face is horribly broke out again. I have pustules _all over my chin_ and _above my lip_ and _my forehead_ is red and inflamed. This has all happened in _a timeframe of 2-3 weeks_ and I'm very _depressed_ about it. I'm trying to figure out what went wrong and why my acne is so bad. I'm not really doing anything differently than I was before, so I have to assume it has something to do with _going to university_.

＊＊＊＊＊

---

[14] Comment posted at "University and Acne?" by PurplGrind at Acne.org, Sep 26, 2011 (available at www.acne.org/messageboard/topic/304594-university-and-acne/).

Lost in the Hundred Acre Wood[15]

I had breakouts throughout middle school and high school, but it wasn't until I went to college that my acne reached clinical proportions worthy of a visit to a dermatologist. For many of us, going away to college is the first time we move away from home. In situations like mine, it meant leaving a suburban or rural town for a more heavily fluoridated city center.

It can also mean roommates, housemates, exam stress, social stress, cafeteria food, fast food, no food, all-nighters, over-nighters, new boyfriends, ex-boyfriends, and a thousand other factors that shape a new life away from home. In the midst of all this personal upheaval, it can be exceedingly difficult to make out the gorilla. But when I look back at my college experience, I see his footprints clearly and they were on a decisively downward path. At the time, I had no choice but to follow him blindly. I now realize he was leading me on a pathway to *depression*.

College was the first time I distinctly remember having the feeling. It's not that I hated being there or even that I wanted to be anywhere else. It was just the first place I remember continually thinking, "What's the point." The feeling tip-toed into my life sophomore year, but darted out of sight when I studied abroad in West Africa. After I returned to Georgetown senior year, it came into full view for the first time.

I remember my sweet college boyfriend sitting with me on a park bench in D.C., trying to explain how to feel happiness from watching birds take flight over the water. It sounded nice, but I just

---

[15] I didn't realize it until after I wrote this section heading, but this is a brilliant idea. Can you imagine Tigger as one of the Others? Rabbit would be Ben because he's mean. Piglet would be Ethan, Ben's lackey. Kanga would be crazy French lady. And Roo, of course, would be her daughter Alex. I guess the Man in Black could be Eeyore??? The role of Jacob would go to Christopher Robin since he is obviously the one pulling all the strings, plus he can cross over into the real world from the forest world. I hope someone will run with this.

couldn't feel it. He bought me a small African violet plant that made me feel hopeful for some unidentified reason and a stuffed hippopotamus, which I admit I still cried into at night as a naval officer years later.

Crying at night was nothing new. In high school, I remember talking with the other girls on the cheerleading squad when one of them casually mentioned that she cried herself to sleep every night for absolutely no good reason. A bunch of us nodded our heads. Yep, that's normal. No cause for concern. We're girls. We cry. That's what we do. We all cry ourselves to sleep at night, and we all get acne.

If you visit the American Academy of Dermatology (AAD) webpage on tips for managing acne, you might notice something peculiar.[16] The tips themselves are not surprising. Wash your skin twice a day. Keep your hands off your face. Don't pick. Don't scrub. Donate your money to dermatologists. Stay out of the sun. But after that, on the bottom of the page and without explanation, there is a link to a suicide hotline. If you click on it, it will lead you to a stock GoDaddy page for a defunct website at suicidehotlines.com. But still. Why is the AAD trying to send people reading about tips for clear skin to a suicide hotline? They don't do that for people searching for tips on acanthosis nigricans (a condition where your skin turns dark and velvety) or alopecia areata (a condition where your hair falls out in patches). Why do they do it for acne?

In 2015, the British Skin Foundation released the results of their largest acne survey to date revealing that out of 2,299 respondents, over 20 percent contemplated or attempted suicide.[17]

The link between suicide and acne has long been documented in the medical literature. In a 1998 article published in the *British Journal of Dermatology*, researchers studied 480 patients with dermatological disorders and found those with mild to moderate acne

---

[16] www.aad.org/dermatology-a-to-z/diseases-and-treatments/a---d/acne/tips

[17] "Over Half of Acne Sufferers Experience Verbal Abuse from Friends and Family Due to Their Condition." British Skin Foundation Press Release, 2015.

experienced more suicidal thoughts than patients with atopic dermatitis, alopecia areata, or psoriasis covering up to 30 percent of their body.[18] The study excluded patients with cystic acne like mine, even though it is not uncommon. Other researchers report depression is two to three times more prevalent in acne patients than in the general population, and that women with acne, especially those over 36 years of age, experience depression over twice as often as men with acne.[19]

The experts most often point to two contributing factors to explain the link between acne and depression. One of the factors is stress. In the title of a 2014 article published in the *Archives of Dermatological Research*, the authors pose a promising question: "Could adult female acne be associated with modern life?"[20] Their review notes the higher risks of depression among women and aims to establish a connection between the stress of the modern daily routine, sleep deprivation, and the recent increase in late-onset female acne.

It is true that college and the average work/life routine are stressful and that stress plays an undeniable role in health. On multiple occasions when I was particularly stressed over exams, I developed painful canker sores inside the sides of my mouth. (Could this be another indicator of fluoride toxicity?) But that only happened to me during exams at Georgetown or in the military. I never experienced stress-induced canker sores during graduate school in unfluoridated Scotland.

The other common explanation for the link between depression and acne is low self-esteem. This one is so intuitive it is difficult to think past it. When you have ugly eruptions plainly visible on your face, it's only natural to feel self conscious when interacting with other

---

[18] Gupta, Gupta, "Depression and suicidal ideation in dermatology patients with acne, alopecia areata, atopic dermatitis and psoriasis." British Journal of Dermatology, vol. 139, 1998, pp. 846–850.

[19] Uhlenhake, Elizabeth et al. "Acne vulgaris and depression: a retrospective examination." *Journal of Cosmetic Dermatology*, Mar 2010.

[20] Albuquerque, R.G.R. et al. "Could adult female acne be associated with modern life." *Archives of Dermatological Research*, vol. 306, 2014, pp. 683–688.

people. Few of us tend to react otherwise. In 1948, researchers published the first study examining the psychological impact of acne and concluded, "There is no single disease which causes more psychic trauma, more maladjustment between parents and children, more general insecurity and feelings of inferiority, and greater sums of psychic suffering than does acne vulgaris."[21] That is a powerful statement for a common skin condition known to come and go with time. There is one unproven word in their conclusion that completely changes our interpretation of what is going on with acne psychologically. If you reread their statement slowly you might notice it. (I will give you a hint—it's seven words in.)

The adage that "correlation does not imply causation" is a central concept in statistics and intelligence analysis alike. The principle is perhaps best illustrated in a spoof article on Bloomberg Business where the author depicts a graph correlating the rise of Facebook with the yield on 10-year government bonds in Greece.[22] He also shows how the U.S. Housing Price Index (HPI) mimics the increase in babies named Ava and how variations in the murder rate in New York state over time are a perfect match for the topography of an identified mountain range.

No matter how many studies show a connection between acne and stress, acne and depression, or even between acne and low self-esteem, these statistics cannot show *causality*. As with Cordain and his pseudo Star Wars lexicon, medical researchers often give in to the temptation to dive into scientific literature and reverse engineer a mechanism to show causality after a correlation has been established in the physical world. Their stories usually involve a lot of big words and microscopic characters which sound very convincing, but the rule stands. Correlation does not even *imply* causation. It is just as possible

---

[21] Sulzberger, M.B., Zaidens, S.H., "Psychogenic factors in dermatological disorders." *Medical Clinics of North America*, vol. 32, 1948, pp. 669-672.

[22] Chandrasekaran, Vali. "Correlation or Causation?" *Bloomburg Business*, Dec 1, 2011.

that acne, feelings of low self-esteem, and depression are all caused by an outside factor yet to be identified.

This is where your dual role as researcher and research subject really comes in handy. You don't need to interpret carefully worded questionnaires or quantify the varying levels of suicide-ness to determine the details of your emotional state. You know your emotions in a way psychologists, psychiatrists, psychotherapists, dermatologists, dentists, or any other -ists in existence ever could. You know the times you felt depressed—you were there. You know all the nuances of the dark thoughts that swim around your emotional states. You know the times you felt optimistic and carefree. And only *you* know the times you cried alone in a dark room wishing to fall asleep and not wake up.

My dark room was my bedroom in Newport, Rhode Island. There was so much going on in my life at the time, the idea that my depression was caused by my acne, let alone by low self-esteem from acne, never entered my mind. I was not happy about going into the military and felt tricked into the predicament by my parents who suggested I should at least take advantage of the first year of my full ROTC scholarship and then cancel without penalty if I decided the military was not right for me. Their proposal sounded reasonable enough, but I didn't realize that canceling the scholarship would mean dropping out of Georgetown, so I stayed even though military service did not appeal to me as a career.

The other major factor in my dark mood was the effect moving to Rhode Island had on my relationship with my college boyfriend—my first love and best friend—who was offered a dream job in New York City after graduation. We somehow held on in Newport and stayed together a couple years longer, but my tumultuous time in Rhode Island was the beginning of the downward trend of our relationship.

Wait a minute. What page is this? I feel like we might be too far into a science-y book without at least including a chart, so in case I can't get a publisher to include illustrations in the finished version of this book, I will now describe some charts for you here. If I were to look back over my life and plot my mood on a chart, it would look similar to a chart of the extent of my acne, which in turn would look similar to a chart of the amount of fluoride I was exposed to through the public water supply. I could use the same chart to demonstrate the times I experienced low points in my personal relationships and the whiteness of my tongue (more on that in a minute). My point is that several of these factors line up in correlation, not necessarily causation, and that a future publisher is getting a pretty darn good deal on a one-size-fits-all chart.[23]

The months I spent in Newport after graduation were my rock bottom. When I left, my mood steadily improved from "make it stop" back up to "what's the point" before hovering over "Melissa, just get through this" and finally reaching "maybe life will be okay after all someday far off in the future."

When I left the U.S. for Tunisia and Scotland, I started to feel good moods more regularly and without effort, unlike any time I could remember. I was sitting on a bench in St. Andrews (if you haven't noticed this yet, sitting on benches bestows unexplained mystical powers—try it, you'll see) when I very clearly realized that my life up to that point felt like a marathon, and I was exhausted from running it. I decided on that very bench that I was not going to let my life continue this way. I was going to stop running and start finding happiness in *this* moment. And I did.

By the end of my time in Scotland, I had outgrown crying myself to sleep at night. I never cried at all anymore. Life was naturally exciting, and I was genuinely happy to be here.

I was shocked when I returned to the United States and my mood immediately plunged into murky but familiar waters. I had no reason to be apathetic about life. I was in love with my dream man

---

[23] Turns out my publisher (aka, me) did not want to jack up the price of this book by including color images. Instead, you can view the chart at ProjectFree.Me/Chart.

who came as a package deal with my dream dog. I had just completed a Fulbright to the United Kingdom, an honor I never imagined I would achieve. And I was living rent-free in my favorite place on earth, the magical sunny kingdom of South Florida. I knew things weren't right when I lost interest in food. I still ate it, but it all seemed so boring and pointless. Rib eye, crab legs, summer berries. Blah. Normally I would feel at least a little sparkle of excitement with simple pleasures like these, but now everything just felt flat.

My boyfriend was the one who suggested maybe my acne was the cause of my depression. I didn't think so. Acne never bothered me like that before. All the other times I had acne I was depressed for *real* reasons. "You seem saddest on the days when your acne is the worst," he pointed out. It was true. Was I subconsciously so upset about my acne that it made me *lose all interest in life*? Could that happen without my approval? Doesn't the conscious me have a say?

I might have started to believe that acne was causing my depression if not for a few gorilla hairs left at the scene. (You should probably know, I thought about writing gorilla droppings there but it sounded crude so I didn't, even though gorilla droppings would be more descriptive and just as apropos.)

As I mentioned earlier, along with my graduate degree in International Security, I had officially started my master's in Health Nuttery while studying abroad in Scotland. By the time I moved back to Florida, I was doing a few things that we in the health nuttery field commonly refer to as "woo-woo health stuff" such as sleeping in total darkness in an attempt to regulate my hormones. The practice involved taking my oral temperature every morning before I got out of bed. It's normal for a woman's waking temperature to be lower before ovulation, but on some days it was remarkably lower than others, close to 97.0 degrees Fahrenheit. I noticed on days like this when my waking temperature was especially low, my mood was at its lowest point, too.

This observation alone could have been written off as a

coincidence, but there was another sign that told me something systemic was going on with my depression. Multiple times after having a really low day, I noticed white marks on my fingernails a day or two later. I've had similar white spots on my nails off and on my whole life, but these were so pronounced and the timing so suspicious that I decided to ask Internet about them.

I came across a Q&A from Andrew Weil, a popular Harvard-trained medical doctor who walks the line between conventional and alternative approaches to health.[24] A reader asked him if the spots are indicative of a mineral deficiency. Weil pulls a common medical doctor tactic by first demonstrating his expertise on the subject (you've probably seen this one before) by busting out some fancy Greek caveman talk to explain that white spots on fingernails are referred to in the medical field as leukonychia, which according to my trusty Greek caveman dictionary (it's Google) translates back into English as the name of the great Native American spirit ghost, "White Nail."

Weil goes on to explain that the marks are usually caused by us crazy knuckleheads knocking our hands on random junk and forgetting about it, or maybe it was a rough manicure or a reaction to nail polish (you know, girl stuff). He closes his expert advice by dispelling some rumors that are making the rounds amongst us kids these days. It is a myth that leukonychia is caused by calcium deficiency, zinc deficiency, or Hellman's mayonnaise. "I'm not making this up," he attests. He sounds serious about that last part, so I believe him.

But the rest of his explanation about the origins of white marks on fingernails did not resonate with my experience of them. Why did I get pronounced white spots on my nails when my mood flatlined and my face broke out? Why didn't I get them in Scotland? Why do some people get white marks on their nails and others do not? I wondered

[24] Weil, Andrew. "Worried About White Spots on Fingernails?" Q&A Library at drweil.com, Feb 11, 2005 (available at www.drweil.com/drw/u/QAA350576/white-spots-on-fingernails.html as of May 2016).

why Weil was so confident in his assessment of the causes of leukonychia. I wondered why doctors are confident in their assessment of anything—how do they know what they *think* they know?

I couldn't envision Weil ever taking the time or effort to test his theories on fingernails in the real world. His explanation seemed like a mashup of the one I read on Wikipedia and one written seven months before Weil's article by a mystery commenter known only as The Geek. The latter debunked the Hellman's mayo myth and was posted in an online forum (pinky swear be damned) at SalonGeek, the world's largest community of salon professionals dedicated to open discussion, personal development and powerful passion for the industry we love.[25]

The white marks on my fingernails reminded me of something. I went to my thinking spot to think, think, think. Ah, I remembered. When I took fluoride pills as a child while my teeth were forming, it showed up as bright white spots on my tooth enamel. Could the same thing be happening with my fingernails? I asked Internet about "fluoride and leukonychia" but she was uncharacteristically quiet on the topic—prolly thought I was showing off.

Then I asked her about "fluoride and fingernails" and she offered a 1999 study by researchers at the Medical College of Georgia who measured fingernail clippings to see if they can be used as a biomarker for subchronic exposure to fluoride.[26] They found that a month of increased fluoride intake resulted in significant increases in fluoride concentrations of fingernail clippings after a lag time of approximately 3.5 months. I was onto something. I asked Internet, "Real quick, how long does it take for fingernails to grow from nail bed to tip." She answered via Wikipedia: 3 months, at least.

---

[25] See "My Big Fat Greek Leukonychia" posted by The Geek, Jul 12, 2004 (available at www.salongeek.com/threads/my-big-fat-greek-leukonychia.6245/).

[26] Whitford, G.M., "Fingernail fluoride: a method for monitoring fluoride exposure." Caries Research, vol. 33, issue 6, Nov-Dec 1999, pp. 462-467.

The white marks on my nails, my low waking temperature, my acne, my depression, and my consumption of fluoride were all correlated. There was evidence that fluoride could be *causing* the white marks on my nails, and I was already vetting the idea it was causing my acne. I formed a testable hypothesis: if fluoride was the cause of my low waking temperature and my depression, then limiting fluoride in my diet should increase my waking temperature and get rid of my depression. The white marks on my fingernails, along with my acne, should disappear for good, too.

I steadily tested my hypothesis over the next few years, and that is exactly what happened. Now that I know how to limit my fluoride exposure, I don't have acne, I don't have white marks on my fingernails, and I don't have depression. Am I just knocking my hands around less and not using them to pick at my bacteria-laden face? Is my life that much better than it was a few years ago that it's now effortless to be happy?

Life is still stressful. I still work long hours, I have an arduous commute and a lot of work-related travel, there's drama with my family, and I'm putting all my free time into writing this book. But clear skin comes naturally for me now and so does happiness. Here's my secret: *that is how it should be when you're not being poisoned.*

*****

HomeBoundGypsy writes at "Depression & Acne" on Acne.org:[27] Whenever *my face is at it's worst,* although I try not to, *I become depressed.* I believe there's a link there. How many of you would say you have been or are in a depression, because of your acne, or is acne related?

> **Blehin replies:** Of course acne can cause depression ...

> **junior11 replies:** It might be true cause *i got depression before the acne.* But things were getting a bit better and then came the acne. Why do you think it might be related?

> **o_Adam_o replies:** isnt it more like, acne effects you in your daily life.. or maybe you think it does, and then you get depressed about it.. or somthing

> **Vicious Lyss replies:** I've never been depressed about acne by itself... I mean, I know it's possible. But I haven't. I have, though, been depressed from other stuff. *Life sucks.*

HomeBoundGypsy writes: That's what I was wondering... does anybody escape depression while having acne? It seems that very few people are fortunate enough to not experience depression because of their acne.

> **whoalisa replies:** I've been *severely depressed* while having acne, but the acne was in no way the cause of my depression. Correlated, maybe. Cause, certainly not.

> **SAK replies:** I'm pretty much at *rock bottom* because of my acne. Quite *suicidal,* actually, even though I feel stupid about feeling that way. *Not leaving the house* isn't enough for me to feel more secure anymore.

---

[27] Comments posted at "Depression & Acne" by HomeBoundGypsy at Acne.org, Nov 1, 2009 (available at www.acne.org/messageboard/topic/252388-depression-acne/).

Chapter 42[28]

Now this is where our story really gets exciting; we have cause for a *second* chart. And not just any chart. We need the mother of all science charts. The periodic table of the elements. Preferably in rainbow. I've never had a book published before, but I feel like publishing people complain about charts and illustrations and such and how expensive they are, so I'm just going to close my eyes and make a wish to the publishing fairy that a second chart—a radiantly multicolored periodic table—appears magically above this paragraph by the time you read it. Or below, whatever. Did it work?[29]

Looking at the periodic table above (fingers crossed!), you will see the F for fluorine at the top of the second to last column on the right. It sits at the head of a group of elements called halogens which are displayed in... pink? The halogen group consists of fluorine, chlorine, bromine, iodine, and astatine. The name halogen means "salt-producing" and was given to this group because of their tendency to react with metals to produce a wide range of salts, including calcium fluoride (a mineral that spawned the word fluorescence), sodium chloride (common table salt) and potassium iodide (what they add to salt to make it "iodized").

To the right of the halogens—silver, please—is a group of elements called the noble gases. This group consists of helium, neon, argon, krypton, xenon, and radon and was given the name noble gases because they do not like to mingle with others. They used to be called inert gases, but scientists later observed that on very rare occasions noble gases can bond with other elements, mostly fluorine because of its extremely high reactivity.

---

[28] If you ask Internet, "what is the answer to life?" she will tell you it's 42. Go ahead. Try it and see: www.google.com/search?q=what+is+the+answer+to+life. (This is foreshadowing for chapter six. I can't wait until you get there!)

[29] Melissa, we are self-publishing here so *no*. Maybe in the ebook edition. But you can post a beautiful periodic table at ProjectFree.Me/Chemistry. Deal?

About a century ago, serious scientists like chemists and physicists realized the number of electrons in the outer shell was a governing factor in how elements bond with each other and their level of reactivity. The reason for the unusual chemical stability of the noble gases is because they each have a full octet of electrons in their outer shell (except for helium who has to be unique and, like a certain heavyweight boxer we know, is clearly overcompensating for his tiny voice). Scientists concluded that all elements are continually trying to reach the stable state that comes with having eight electrons in their outer shell, as epitomized by the noble gases.

The entire periodic table is set up around this principle, with elements in each column forming groups that reflect the number of electrons in their outer shells. Group 1, headed by hydrogen (H) located all the way on the left, only has one electron in their outer shell. This lonely electron is easily lost, explaining why elements in this group are so unstable and why you should always fill your blimps with helium, a noble gas, instead of hydrogen, from whence the term H-bomb is derived.

Continuing along our periodic table from left to right, elements in each column increase their outer electron count by one. So Group 2, headed by beryllium (Be), has two outer electrons. The "transition metals" in Groups 3 to 12 get weird with this so scientists try to tuck them all in together and then continue along like nothing strange happened with Group 13, the boron (B) group, which has three electrons in their outer shell, etc. If you keep counting, you'll see that Group 17, the halogens, has an outer shell with seven electrons—so close to nobility! Fluorine, more than any of the other halogens, wants to be king *so bad* he'll do whatever it takes. All he needs is one more lousy electron in his outer shell and the kingdom is his. (Pause here for dramatic effect.) This missing electron is what makes fluorine so unstable.

Fluorine is more reactive than other halogens because it is the lightest. Elements at the top of their group in the periodic table have the smallest atomic weight, a property that increases as you descend down each column. I'm telling you all this not because I need an excuse for a publisher to include THE PRETTIEST CHEMISTRY CHART EVER in my book, but so you have a better understanding of what it means when people make the claim that fluoride is the most reactive element on the planet.

Chemists nicknamed fluorine "the tiger of chemistry" because it kills so many overconfident chemists in the lab. Dentists, on the other hand, like to point out that fluoride is a naturally occurring natural mineral, that it exists naturally in virtually all natural water supplies, and that nature herself chose it as the thirteenth most abundant natural element in the earth's natural crust, naturally. But now you know there is more to the story. Fluoride's abundance explains why it is the byproduct of so many big industries and its high reactivity explains why it causes so many damaging health effects throughout the human body.

Government bodies like the U.S. Public Health Service (PHS) have been caught passing notes in class[30] with statements like "Fluoride: An Essential Mineral Nutrient."[31] Contrary to PHS rumors, nutrients are commonly defined as biochemical substances that provide energy or building material for the survival and growth of a living organism. A nutrient is considered essential if it must be obtained from external sources. This is not the case with fluoride.

When essential nutrients are restricted from the diet, predictable side effects develop. For example, if you can't sleep at night, your skin turns pale and mysteriously starts blistering at the thought of sunshine, blood drips from your swollen mouth, and you become aggressive to the point of insanity, you might need to beef up

---

[30] Little Known Fact: PHS was the actual initials for my high school.

[31] For example, see "Fluoride: An Essential Mineral Nutrient" by the U.S. Public Health Service, Jun 1974 (available at ProjectFree.Me/Fluoride-Rumor).

on your B3 intake.[32] There is no evidence that restricting fluoride in the diet has any negative effects on the body whatsoever, even on teeth. Therefore it is not considered an essential nutrient. To quote Lorde, one of the most popular kids in class, "So there."

In fact, there is little evidence that fluoride is even a nutrient. As you will learn in the next chapter, there are a lot of foods in the modern diet that contain significant amounts of fluoride, but in the majority of cases—tea leaves being the prime exception—the fluoride found in our food supply is not naturally occurring. Most of it comes from pesticides and from the pollution of phosphate fertilizer plants that dental devotees insist we all use to drink, bathe, and wash our underwear (so creepy).

Even fluoride that occurs naturally in some water sources is more a matter of geology than biology. If the water happens to run through fluoride-heavy rocks such as cryolite or bauxite, then it too will contain high amounts of fluoride. This is why deep water wells are more likely to contain significant doses of fluoride than most spring water sources. People in certain parts of India, China, and elsewhere suffer severe health consequences because of naturally occurring fluoride in their water supply.[33]

Mother Nature gave us a big clue about the place of fluoride in the human diet when she installed what one study in the *British Medical Journal* describes as "a physiological plasma-milk barrier" that prevents fluoride from being passed to breastfeeding infants.[34] If fluoride is helpful for growing strong teeth, why does Mother Nature

---

[32] Hampl, J. S., and W.S. Hampl. "Pellagra and the Origin of a Myth: Evidence from European Literature and Folklore." *Journal of the Royal Society of Medicine,* vol. 90, issue 11, 1997, pp. 636–639.

[33] For more information, see Connett, Michael. "Skeletal Fluorosis in India and China" Fluoride Action Network, May 2012 (available at www.fluoridealert.org/studies/skeletal_fluorosis05/).

[34] Ekstrand, J., Boreus, L.O., and de Chateau, P. "No Evidence of Transfer of Fluoride from Plasma to Breast Milk." *British Medical Journal (Clinical research ed.)* 283.6294, 1981, pp. 761–762.

withhold it from us at the time we would need it most? Knowing her, that doesn't sound like something she would do.

While there is no evidence that indicates fluoride is an essential nutrient, another member of the halogen group, iodine, clearly is. Individuals with severe iodine deficiency develop an enlarged thyroid gland visible as a swollen protrusion around their neck, a condition known as goiter. In severe cases, a lack of iodine can result in cretinism, a condition characterized by the lack of both physical and mental development.

A less recognizable sign of iodine deficiency is *hypo*thyroidism, a common disorder of the endocrine system where the thyroid gland does not produce enough thyroid hormone. Symptoms of hypothyroidism include dry skin, cold hands, *low body temperature*, fatigue, irritability, mental haziness, constipation, and weight gain. It is worth noting that women with melasma, the dark facial pigment I developed when using benzoyl peroxide for my acne, are found to be four times more likely to have hypothyroidism.[35] The experts disagree on how many people in the United States have underactive thyroid glands, but they do agree the number is well into the millions and that the majority are women. Harvard researchers predict one in five women will develop hypothyroidism by age 60.[36]

Iodine and fluorine are located at opposite ends of the halogen group. Since iodine is the heaviest of the halogens found in the human body (and the heaviest of all elements needed by living organisms), it loses out to other halogens that compete for the same receptors. When we have high amounts of fluoride in our diets, especially when iodine is lacking, our bodies absorb fluoride where they would normally absorb iodine. For example, until the 1950s, doctors in Europe and South America prescribed fluoride to *reduce* thyroid activity in patients

---

[35] Lute, R.J., "Association of melasma with thyroid autoimmunity and other thyroidal abnormalities and their relationship to the origin of the melasma." *Journal of Clinical Endocrinology and Metabolism*, vol. 61, issue 1, 1985, pp. 28-31.

[36] "When Depression Starts in the Neck," Harvard Mental Health Letter, Jul 1, 2011.

with *hyper*thyroidism.[37] They found that a dose as low as 2 to 5 milligrams per day over a period of a few months decreased thyroid activity in their patients.

Fluoride's propensity to displace iodine explains why fluoride causes such a wide variety of negative health effects. Discussions of dietary iodine tend to focus on the thyroid gland, but iodine is needed throughout the glandular system, including in the breasts, ovaries (which also produce thyroid hormone), pancreas, thymus, salivary glands, etc. Fluoride competes with iodine for receptors in these glands, as well. In the late 1990s, Jennifer Luke, a doctoral candidate in the United Kingdom, dissected eleven human pineal glands and discovered that calcified portions of the gland contain the highest concentrations of fluoride in the human body—up to 21,000 ppm.[38] The pineal gland secretes melatonin and helps regulate the seasonal and circadian rhythms of the body.

As with acne, there is a documented link between hypothyroidism and depression. A 2006 study published in the *American Journal of Psychiatry* examined 142 adult patients with major depressive disorder who did not achieve remission even after two optimally delivered trials of antidepressant medications.[39] The study found that 25 percent of test patients who received a thyroid hormone supplement went into remission for their depression after just 14 weeks. The clear role of iodine and the thyroid gland in mental health could at least partially explain the correlation between acne (aka fluoroderma) and depression. It also sheds light on the mysterious role played by hormones in the development of acne. Dermatologists,

---

[37] Galletti, Pierre M.. Joyet, Gustave."Effect of Fluorine on Thyroidal Iodine Metabolism in Hyperthyroidism," *Journal of Clinical Endocrinology*, vol. 18, 1958, pp. 1102-1110.

[38] Luke, J. et al., "The Effect of Fluoride on the Physiology of the Pineal Gland." Ph.D. Thesis, University of Surrey, Guildford, 1997.

[39] Nierenberg, Andrew A. et al., "A Comparison of Lithium and T 3 Augmentation Following Two Failed Medication Treatments for Depression: A STAR*D Report," *The American Journal of Psychiatry*, vol. 163, issue 9, Sep 2006, pp. 1519-1530.

teenagers, and women with eyes and brains have noticed a correlation between acne and hormonal fluctuations caused by puberty, menstruation, birth control pills, pregnancy, etc. The official explanation doesn't go much beyond the idea that certain hormones make your face shiny,[40] but there must be more to the story than that.

The human body does not restrict its use of iodine to the endocrine system. Concentrations of iodine are also found in cerebrospinal fluid and throughout the brain.[41] When Phyllis Mullenix, the prominent toxicologist and fluoridation pagan discussed in the previous chapter, began studying fluoride, the existing scientific literature led her to believe fluoride, unlike iodine, does not cross the blood-brain barrier. But she was suspicious of previous studies because they administered fluoride via injection and then measured fluoride content of the brain an hour later.[42] To more accurately reflect the way humans are chronically exposed to fluoride in the water supply, she conducted an experiment by giving 532 rats fluoridated water and then measuring the fluoride content of their brains several weeks later.[43]

---

[40] According to information presented at the American Academy of Dermatology's 70th Annual Meeting by Bethanee Jean Schlosser, MD, PhD, FAAD, assistant professor of dermatology and director of Women's Skin Health at Northwestern University, Feinberg School of Medicine, the key hormonal factor in understanding acne is as follows: "Androgens, the male hormones present in both men and women, can contribute to acne flares by overstimulating the oil glands and altering the development of skin cells that line hair follicles in the skin." As cited at "Hormonal factors key to understanding acne in women," AAD.org, Mar 16, 2012.

[41] Adrasi, E., "Iodine concentration in different human brain parts." *Analytical and Bioanalytical Chemistry*, Nov 13, 2003.

[42] Connett, Paul. "Fluoride & the Brain: An Interview with Dr. Phyllis Mullenix," October 18, 1997 (available at www.fluoridealert.org/content/mullenix-interview/).

[43] You might be surprised when you see that the rats in Mullenix's study received water containing fluoride at 100 ppm. This confused the dentists, too. Because of her training in toxicology, Mullenix knew to begin her studies by using animal doses that produce a level of fluoride in the plasma equivalent to that found in humans drinking fluoridated water and using fluoridated dental treatments. Her efforts to conduct followup studies were not funded and she was dismissed from her position. Mullenix, Phyllis J., "Neurotoxicity of sodium fluoride in rats," *Neurotoxicology and Teratology*, vol. 17, issue 2, Mar-Apr 1995, pp. 169–177.

Mullenix and her team were shocked when they discovered major accumulations of fluoride in every section of the brain. Their studies show that rats with post-natal exposure to fluoride exhibit symptoms of *hypo*activity while those with pre-natal exposure to fluoride exhibit symptoms of *hyper*activity. This evidence prompted the growing concern that fluoride could be a contributing factor in the prevalence of Attention Deficit Hyperactivity Disorder (ADHD) in the United States, a claim supported by recent demographic studies comparing rates of ADHD and fluoridation.[44]

In a 2012 meta-analysis of the scientific literature on fluoride neurotoxicity, Harvard researchers reviewed 27 studies on the subject and found that all but one showed a significant link between higher levels of fluoride in the water supply and reduced IQ.[45] As Caroline Martinez, a pediatrician and researcher at Mt. Sinai Hospital in New York, explains, "Fluoride appears to fit in with a pattern of other trace elements such as lead, methylmercury, arsenic, cadmium and manganese—adverse effects of these have been documented over time at exposures previously thought to be 'low' and 'safe.'"[46]

These are just a few of the adverse health effects caused by fluoride exposure. The full list is much more extensive because every cell, organ, and tissue in the human body evolved using iodine—an abundant element in ocean water—in place of fluoride, which modern industry has unearthed in unnatural proportions from deep within the earth's crust. I have not even touched on fluoride's role in arthritis[47],

---

[44] Malin, Ashley J., Till, Christine, "Exposure to fluoridated water and attention deficit hyperactivity disorder prevalence among children and adolescents in the United States: an ecological association," *Environmental Health,* vol. 14, issue 17, 2015.

[45] Choi, Anna L. et al. "Developmental Fluoride Neurotoxicity: A Systematic Review and Meta-Analysis," *Environmental Health Perspective*, vol. 120, issue 10, 2012, pp. 1362-1368. For more studies on fluoride neurotoxicity, see www.fluoridealert.org/studies/brain01/.

[46] As quoted in "Water Fluoridation Linked to Higher ADHD Rates" by Douglas Main, *Newsweek*, Mar 10, 2015.

[47] See fluoridealert.org/issues/health/arthritis/.

rheumatoid arthritis,[48] bone fractures,[49] certain types of cancer,[50] infertility,[51] kidney disease,[52] fibromyalgia,[53] and many other debilitating conditions that plague our industrialized society. Even though you are likely reading this book because you want to heal your acne, acne is not the root problem. Like these other disorders, it is a symptom of chronic fluoride poisoning, a term I don't use for dramatic effect but because it is appropriate.

When you look at your acne as a symptom of a larger story, you will have a better vantage point for observing the full picture of how fluoride is affecting your body. When my fluoroderma was at its worst, acne was not the only physical sign something was very wrong. In addition to depression, I often had a thick oily residue in my hair. When I went for acupuncture, the doctor remarked on the whiteness of my tongue and called in her assistant to show her. In Traditional Chinese Medicine, a thick white coating on the tongue represents excess dampness in the body. In addition, my breath smelled bad even though I brushed and flossed more and made an extra effort to stay well hydrated.

Since I'm putting it all out there at this point, I might as well tell you I had bad body odor, too. When I lived acne-free in Senegal, I forgot to pack my special hypoallergenic deodorant so I went without it for nearly a year in one of the hottest countries on earth. I might have been sweaty, but I never remember smelling bad and my roommate swore I didn't, either. In Delray Beach where the water was heavily fluoridated, I smelled bad sitting in the air conditioning all day.

---

[48] See fluoridealert.org/studies/arthritis03/.

[49] See fluoridealert.org/issues/health/bone-fracture/.

[50] See fluoridealert.org/issues/health/cancer/.

[51] See fluoridealert.org/issues/health/fertility/.

[52] See fluoridealert.org/issues/health/kidney/.

[53] See ncbi.nlm.nih.gov/pubmed/18179362.

Speaking of hypoallergenic deodorant, skin sensitivities are another potential indicator of fluoride toxicity. The reason I couldn't simply purchase a new deodorant when I forgot mine in Senegal is because in high school I developed a severe skin sensitivity to most deodorants. I also had skin reactions to laundry detergents, fabric softeners, shaving cream, body scrubs, the little moisturizing strips on razors, and probably a bunch of other chemical products I was never able to identify. These are the kinds of little quirks you might not bother mentioning to doctors and if you did they would have no idea what to tell you. But whether the clues provided by your health conditions are big or small, they help tell the story of your body in a way only *you* might ever be likely to decipher.

For example, when I moved to Jacksonville, Florida, I developed a recurring rash on my right forearm. It came and went many times, but I couldn't figure out the cause. I asked a military doctor about it at a routine physical. He in turn asked if I used one of those poof things in the shower. I said I did, and he told me I was probably scrubbing too hard. I didn't say anything at the time, but something in his answer made me wonder how closely he was paying attention during his poof class at medical school. My incessant intelligence analyst brain wondered why the rash only appeared on my right arm. Wouldn't I naturally scrub harder on my left arm since I am right handed? And why didn't the rash appear elsewhere I scrubbed with my left arm since I was likely scrubbing those areas with the same intensity? (See how annoying intelligence analyst brains can be?) I left Jacksonville for nearly a year during which time the rash never came back, but when I returned to Jacksonville it quickly made a reappearance.

Now that I know more about how the human body responds to fluoride and my particular history with it, I can easily develop my own hypothesis about the mystery rash on my arm. Perhaps the location of the rash is because I broke my right forearm when I was in kindergarten and the bone bioaccumulated additional fluoride during the healing process since that was the same timeframe when I was ingesting fluoride pills. Perhaps the timing of the rash is because I purchased a cheap mattress in Jacksonville from a mattress discount warehouse which I suspect sprayed their piles of unwrapped mattresses (it was seriously discounted) with either fluoride-based pesticides or bromine-based flame-retardants. Bromine is another dangerous halogen we'll discuss in an upcoming chapter.

I didn't figure out the mattress connection until it went into storage for a couple years and then ended up in a guest room in my current house. When we were painting our master bedroom, my husband and I slept in the guest room and after a two year absence, the mystery rash again made a reappearance. It was the first time I ever saw it outside of Jacksonville so I knew the cause was something I brought with me. A doctor would never have been able to put all these clues together, but because they involve small details of my everyday life, I am naturally the expert in such matters.

And so are you.

*****

Happily Ever After

There are a lot of blank pages we still need to fill before we reach the end of our story. An important part of any analysis is trying to identify and articulate your known intelligence gaps. With regard to my analysis of fluoroderma, one intel gap is that I don't know what percentage of acne in the general population is caused by fluoride. But I suspect it is a significant portion.

When George Waldbott, the renowned allergist and early fluoridation pagan, published his series of case reports and double-blind studies in the 1950s, he found that one percent of the population experienced hypersensitivity to ingested fluoride from the water supply.[54] His findings were replicated by the largest government-funded clinical trial of fluoride supplements, which confirmed that one percent of children given a daily 1 mg fluoride tablet—the amount contained in one liter of water fluoridated at the recommended level—exhibited adverse reactions such as eczema, atopic dermatitis, and hives.[55]

You might be wondering why the government funded a critical study of fluoridation, but there is a completely logical explanation. They didn't realize that is what they were doing. The U.S. Public Health Service ceased funding for the study prior to its 10-year target date because they thought it was supposed to be a study "to determine the efficacy (in preventing caries) of the addition of measured doses of fluoride salts to pregnant women and children." They were not interested in funding studies on the adverse health effects of fluoride. The study continued anyway and the results were published in the *Journal of Dental Medicine* in 1961 after fourteen years of investigation.[56]

If one percent of the population in 1950s America was hypersensitive to fluoride, in the absence of contemporary follow-up studies, we can only extrapolate what that statistic might be today. We have endured seventy years of public water fluoridation, fluoride-based pesticides are pervasive in the food supply, and we live with fluoridated teeth and bones inherited from our parents not through genetics but through the cultural inheritance of a government health system that failed to outsmart industry influence and then got caught

---

[54] For a partial list of Waldbott's publications from the 1950s on fluoride, see ProjectFree.Me/References.

[55] Feltman, R., "Prenatal and postnatal ingestion of fluoride salts: A progress report." *Dental Digest*, vol. 62, 1956, pp. 353-357.

Feltman, R.; Kosel, G. "Prenatal and postnatal ingestion of fluorides – Fourteen years of investigation – Final report." *Journal of Dental Medicine*, vol. 16, 1961, pp. 190-99.

[56] Rorty, J. appendix 1 in *The American Fluoridation Experiment* by F. B. Exner and G.L. Whaleboat, Devin-Adair Company, New York, 1957, pp. 229-241 (as cited by Paul Connett et al, *The Case Against Fluoride*, Chelsea Green Publishing, 2010, p. 129).

up in its own fiction. We have been living with fluoridation for so long, it has literally become a part of who we are. None of us know what our skin—or our society—would look like without it.

In the 1990s, a cunning but unwitting group of Finnish dentists provided a rare glimpse of how the cessation of public water fluoridation would affect the rate of skin conditions in the general population. The town of Kuopio, Finland with 83,000 inhabitants was the only town in the Nordic countries to fluoridate its water supply. After 33 years of anti-fluoridation campaigning that climaxed in bitter local disputes, the City Council finally agreed to discontinue fluoridation in 1992. Dentists at Kuopio University Hospital sensed an opportunity to expose the alleged health complaints associated with fluoride as psychological manifestations of an ignorant populace. They devised a plan to discontinue fluoridation early without informing the public and then to study the occurrence of various symptoms among a group of people who believed that the piped water was still fluoridated even though it was not.

There was little chance the Finnish dentists would see the gorilla in his tutu who was about to dance across the stage.[57] In their study published in a 1997 issue of *Community Dentistry and Oral Epidemiology*, the authors point out their own preconceived bias: "The results obtained were mostly expected and, in our opinion, quite convincing... it seems likely that the prevalence of the symptoms considered in the current study is connected with the psychological rather than with the physical effects of being exposed to fluoridated water." Oh, dentists. Why do you make us do this to you? Let's take a closer look at this one last study before we move on to the next part of our story.

In November when people in Kuopio knew the water was still fluoridated, the dentists sent one thousand surveys asking for recipients to check a box next to a list of 25 symptoms to indicate those they were currently experiencing (acne was not one of the choices). In

---

[57] First author to ever write that line... I called it.

December, they sent another thousand surveys to a separate group of people who were unaware that the amount of fluoride in the water had returned to natural levels three weeks prior. In March, they sent the same survey again to both groups. All recipients were between the ages of 25 and 64, excluding two of the most susceptible demographics. (That's fine. Whatever. Moving on.)

When comparing the differences in the rates of reported symptoms between November when the first group knew the water was fluoridated and December when the second group only thought it was fluoridated, the difference was found to be *highly significant* for one symptom: "other skin rash." Did the dentists focus on this information in the summary of their findings? No, that was not the story they expected—or wanted—to tell. But between pontifications on the psychological antics of anti-fluoridationists, the dentists admit, "The significant decrease in the number of other skin rashes leaves room for speculation [*author note: telling word choice there, no?*], seeming to favor the view that a small segment of the population may have some kind of intolerance to fluoride. This group of people should be studied further [but not by us obviously]." FYI, I added that last part for emphasis.

Furthermore, the entire Kuopio study is based on the dentists' stated assumption that symptoms of chronic fluoride poisoning will pass as quickly as symptoms of acute fluoride poisoning. I'm not a toxicologist so I am relying on my little layman brain here (then again, dentists aren't toxicologists either so...), but I would not assume the symptoms of 30+ years of chronic fluoride poisoning would be completely alleviated after three weeks. Aren't the mechanisms for acute poisoning and chronic poisoning different?

For example, if a child suffers acute fluoride poisoning after accidentally swallowing 0.1 ounces of bubble-gum flavored toothpaste,[58] she would likely experience symptoms of the flu such as

---

[58] See "Acute Fluoride Poisoning from Toothpaste Ingestion" available at www.fluoridealert.org/studies/acute03/.

stomach pain, headaches, nausea, and vomiting that would clear in a few weeks at most. In contrast, a woman in India who is about to develop severe skeletal fluorosis from chronic fluoride poisoning due to fluoride in her water supply would exhibit symptoms of joint pain and stiffness similar to arthritis.[59] No one would expect the symptoms of the pre-fluorosis woman in India to clear after just three weeks or even three months of receiving unfluoridated water.

My most severe fluoroderma flareups lasted up to a month and it took me a few years to figure out how to clear my acne completely. The questions on the Finnish survey were all yes or no. Either you had depression and joint pain from one month to the next, or you did not; there was no room for anything in between.

If you will indulge my analytic tendencies a bit further, it would be insightful to take a moment to make an assessment of our assessments on the health studies we have examined in more detail thus far. You might have noticed a common theme running through our conclusions. In the chocolate bar study, the paleo studies with the Kitavan/Ache/Melbourne participants, the Grand Rapids experiment, and now this Finnish survey, the researchers from all of these efforts got into trouble when they stopped reporting on *what* they were observing and started reporting on *why*. It wasn't the natural world that was steering them wrong, it was their interpretation of it.

Researchers are human (even dentists) and as such are limited by the cognitive traps we all face. My ulterior motivation for looking at these studies with you so closely is to demonstrate that it doesn't take a degree in medicine to put forward a thoughtful assessment of the researchers' conclusions. Scientific literature can look overwhelming with all the sacred words, charts, and statistics, but there is usually enough English for anyone reading this book to follow along with whatever story the authors of scientific studies are telling. With Internet's help, we have the opportunity to add our previously

---

[59] See "Skeletal Fluorosis in India and Its Relevance to the West" available at www.fluoridealert.org/articles/india-fluorosis/.

muffled voices to the dominant conversation on acne and health in general. That is why I've tried to include links to every study I referenced[60]—to encourage you to go to the source and look at the evidence yourself with your unique vantage point, fresh eyes, and your little layman brain. :)

Another intelligence gap is that we do not know if there are other dietary elements that cause acne, and if so how those elements affect the development of fluoroderma. Even if I were the only person in the world who experiences acne from ingested fluoride, my case study would still evidence the fact that acne, at least in certain situations, is caused by diet—a reality most dermatologists refuse to accept. As hard as it is for dermatologists to believe, the existence of even just one case of fluoroderma shows there must be a physical mechanism in place for certain substances that enter your body through your mouth on their way to your stomach to be broken down into smaller components and then somehow circulated to other areas of your body, sometimes ending up all the way back up around your mouth where they started. (Some researchers speculate the existence of such mechanisms and refer to them simply as the digestive and circulatory systems.)

We do not know if other elements use these same mechanisms to cause acne. In *The Hidden Plague*, our fellow health investigator, Tara Grant, describes how she discovered that nightshades, a family of flowering plants that includes tomatoes, potatoes, eggplant, and peppers, among others, were the cause of her acne-like skin condition known as hidradenitis suppurativa. Nightshades contain chemical compounds called alkaloids which evolved as natural pesticides to protect the plants from bugs and predators. Similar to fluoride, some of the strongest evidence of nightshade sensitivity is its connection to

---

[60] In the References .pdf available at **ProjectFree.Me/References**, I tried to include a link to the full text article when possible, but sometimes only abstracts were publicly available. Oftentimes alumni associations or local libraries will enable you to access full text articles online. Check with your alma matter or your local librarian for more information.

arthritis and joint pain.[61] Could it also be a hidden cause of acne? And what is its relation, if any, to fluoride intoxication?

Other signs indicate a connection between acne and additional foods that commonly cause food sensitivities, such as grains, gluten, sugar, soy, and dairy (I have a hypothesis for that last one; will explain soon). The absence of certain elements can cause skin problems, as well. For example, the lack of iodine has a clear effect on skin health as does zinc deficiency. An imbalance of bacteria in the digestive system might also play a role. Our analysis of Cordain's hormonal theory of acne shows how some of these connections can be confused with fluoroderma. Once fluoride is removed from the equation, it will be easier for researchers—including you—to assess any other potential acne culprits.

Which brings us to the most important intelligence gap in our analysis: we do not know the source of *your* acne. I am confident in my assessment that fluoride was the cause of mine, but I do not know if it is causing yours. Our time together has been brief thus far, and you've patiently allowed me to monopolize our whole conversation. You now know all the details of my travel history, my secret depression, even the spots on my fingernails—but I know very little about you. And yet your part in the story of acne is *the most important*. Your experience will help determine if fluoride-induced acne is an anomaly or if my assessment is accurate that acne is a condition of western civilization because of our chronic fluoride intoxication. The ending of our story can only be written by you.

The best way to diagnose fluoroderma is through direct observation of fluoride's effect on your skin. Some people ask me about blood or urine tests to gauge fluoride sensitivity. While those tests do exist, you don't need a test to tell you how your skin reacts to fluoride. You can just look in the mirror. Fluoride tests are not common

---

[61] Childers, N.F.; Margoles, M.D., "An Apparent Relation of Nightshades (Solanaceae) to Arthritis," *Journal of Neurological and Orthopedic Medical Surgery*, vol. 12, 1993, pp. 227-231.

in the United States, and the results would leave a lot of room for interpretation as to their ramifications for your acne. For example, if you measured the amount of fluoride in your urine, it would only show a minuscule picture of what is going on with fluoride in your body. It will not tell you if you have fluoroderma or high amounts of fluoride in your teeth, bones, plasma, or other tissues.

It is not a coincidence that the most effective test for fluoroderma is also the simplest. Like the PHS researchers who tested for fluoride sensitivity by giving children 1 mg of fluoride per day and then observing its effect, once you know the common sources of fluoride in our industrialized life, you can readily observe how your skin reacts after you are exposed to them. Since most people in America are already overwhelmed by fluoride exposure, the safest way to gauge your sensitivity is to start eliminating major sources of fluoride and see if your skin improves. Initially, it is important to look for a reduction in acne rather than a complete elimination as it is difficult to root out hidden sources of fluoride all at once.

An easy way to begin is to stop using fluoridated toothpaste and mouthwash. Non-fluoridated versions are available at any health store. If your fluoroderma is triggered purely by topical contact, then your acne will completely heal with this one simple move. Although dentists and dermatologists rarely mention this, there is a body of scientific literature documenting the causal relationship between topical applications of fluoride and perioral dermatitis,[62] a condition that was never reported prior to the mid-1950s during the early years of fluoridation.[63]

To address the deep cystic welts, you will need to lower the amount of fluoride you are consuming in your diet. You could begin by reducing your consumption of artificially fluoridated drinking

[62] For references and excerpts, see "Hypersensitive Reactions to Topical Fluorides" at the Fluoride Action Network website (available at www.fluoridealert.org/studies/hypersensitivity02/).

[63] Mellette , J. Ramsey, "Perioral Dermatitis," *Journal of the Association of Military Dermatologists,* vol. 9, 1983, pp. 3-8.

water. In Part Two, we will discuss how to determine if your water source is fluoridated and if so, what options are available to reduce your exposure.

If you have masochistic tendencies, you could confirm your fluoroderma in one step by eating a low quality chicken hot dog or wonton soup prepared from a cheap chicken carcass, although I do not recommend it. These were the sources of my most severe fluoroderma flareups and resulted in cystic breakouts a few hours later around my jaw and down the front, back, and sides of my neck. As with humans, chickens are not immune to the bioaccumulation of fluoride from their pesticide-laden food supply.

There is one last intelligence gap I would like to point out. For the most part, throughout my assessment of fluoroderma thus far I've tried to focus on the tangible evidence that shows fluoride is the root cause of acne while refraining from theoretical explanations of *why* fluoride causes acne. As we've seen in our examinations of previous health studies, the *why* can be a much more complicated question to untangle. We know fluoride is a highly reactive element and that it bioaccumulates in various parts of the human body following exposure in unnatural proportions, including in teeth and bones. We know fluoride and iodine are both halogens and that they both have an effect on hormones, particularly thyroid hormones. We also know iodine is essential for healthy skin and mental wellbeing. But why does long-term fluoride ingestion lead to skin eruptions? What exactly is going on inside our bodies that causes fluoride to end up on our faces? I have a theory but I'll save it for a little later.

What I do know is that the *whats* and the *whys* dermatologists have been professing since the advent of dermatology are not a full or even an accurate depiction of the story. Dermatologists still claim that a proximate cause of acne is that we have excess oil on our skin because our oil glands are over-productive. These are such relative terms, "excess" and "over"-productive. Maybe our bodies have good reason to produce extra oil upon certain hormonal cues. Maybe our glands are perfectly-productive under the current circumstances.

Dermatologists describe acne as a disease, but what is a disease *really*? My experience with fluoroderma leads me to believe that acne is not a disease. Our oil glands and our hormones—and our bodies—are not malfunctioning. They are functioning exactly as they should be, given their environment and the raw material provided. Acne is not a disease that needs to be treated. It is a message that needs to be heard. It is nature's way of saying "danger: do not consume." If not for acne, I would not have healed my depression by learning how to avoid fluoride. Each breakout was a signpost, pointing the way back to physical and emotional health.

You are not in a fight against acne. Acne is not the enemy. To quote a wise woman oracle who I was told on good authority knows all the secrets of the universe, we're on each other's team.

PART TWO: AFFECT (*v.*)

4

STOPPING BREAKOUTS BEFORE THEY START

"Took a wrong turn and we
Fell down a rabbit hole...
Didn't they tell us don't rush into things...
Didn't you calm my fears with a Cheshire cat smile...
We found Wonderland,
You and I got lost in it."

—Taylor Swift, *Wonderland*

IF YOU ARE INCLINED TO TRUST HEALTH AUTHORITIES, it can be an unpleasant awakening to realize the CDC is an unwitting Queen of Hearts shouting "off with their heads" while living in a house of cards.

It can be even more disconcerting to learn the cystic welts on your face are caused by common tap water. The everyday world takes on new shades of danger. You start to wonder about the free glass of ice water at a restaurant. Maybe you notice an unsettling feeling as you sink into a warm bath. The double ristretto venti decaf caramel frappuccino from your favorite coffee shop is eyed with new suspicion.[1] Once you suspect fluoride is causing your acne, the world around you doesn't look the same. But it won't always be that way.

Preventing acne should be as effortless for you as it is for a Kitavan. The longterm solution is to end artificial water fluoridation

---

[1] Does Starbucks contain fluoride? To find out, see ProjectFree.Me/Does-Starbucks-Contain-Fluoride.

and demand more responsible use of fluoride-based pesticides (see Appendix: The Plan). But you don't have time right now to move your pawn-self across the whole chessboard for a chance to rewrite the royal decrees. You need to start healing your acne *today*.

Artificial water fluoridation will end—and I predict it will be our generation that makes it happen—but you don't have to wait until then before you can live acne-free. Once you understand where fluoride comes from and how it makes its way into the industrialized food supply, you will know how to choose foods and drinks that are naturally low in fluoride. You will know, for example, that beer and wine can both contain significant amounts of fluoride but for different reasons. More importantly, understanding those reasons elucidates how to choose options that will not contribute to future breakouts.

When I was lying on my couch in Delray Beach with my raw face painted in yogurt, I wished for a computer printout of every factor that was causing my acne. I thought it was an impassible dream at the time,[2] but three years later I realized I was printing its fulfillment when I made a hard copy of an online cheat sheet I created to help other people suffering from fluoroderma. You can download the cheat sheet at **ProjectFree.Me/Fluoride**. (You are going to need it.)

Dentists use the fact that fluoride is found throughout the food supply to demonstrate its safety, but you will soon see the weakness in that argument. At first glance, the list of fluoride sources appears to be a random assortment of foods, drinks, and other arbitrary means of fluoride exposure. But things aren't always as they seem. There is a logic behind the madness, and it is readily deciphered by curious minds.

*****

---

[2] No, I do mean impassible. Nothing's impossible.

The "DRINK ME" Potions

Let's begin at the beginning with fluoridated water and then, as the Red King decrees, we will go until we come to the end and stop.

As I mentioned in Part One, fluoride in water can occur naturally, or it can be added artificially at local water treatment plants. Well water will absorb fluoride naturally if it runs through fluoride-based rock. Since fluoride is the thirteenth most abundant element in the earth's crust, naturally fluoridated water is not an uncommon occurrence. A known fluoride belt stretches from Syria through Jordan, Egypt, Libya, Algeria, Sudan, and Kenya. Another extends from Turkey through Iraq, Iran, Afghanistan, India, northern Thailand, and China.

Deep water wells and those at the foot of high mountains are particularly susceptible to fluoride accumulation, but individual wells throughout the United States and elsewhere have also been found to contain high amounts of fluoride. A 2008 report from the U.S. Geological Survey notes that four percent of sampled wells in the United States exceed the EPA's secondary maximum contaminant level for fluoride of 2.0 ppm.[3]

The CDC recommends having your well water tested for fluoride at least once every three years and urges alternative drinking water sources if the level of fluoride is greater than 2 ppm.[4] Your skin, however, will likely disagree with that number. An amount under 0.1 ppm is more desirable. A survey conducted by Canadian environmental officials found the average fluoride content of fresh surface water such as lakes, rivers and springs to be 0.05 ppm.[5] The

---

[3] See "Private Well Water and Fluoride" (available at www.cdc.gov/fluoridation/faqs/wellwater.htm#q3).

[4] *Ibid.*

[5] Environment Canada. "Inorganic Fluorides: Priority Substances List Assessment Report." Government of Canada, Ottawa, 1993.

average fluoride content of rain water is even lower at 0.008 ppm.[6]

If your residence is connected to a public water municipality, you can confirm the fluoride content by researching the most recent water quality report, also known as consumer confidence reports. All community water systems are required to provide a full water quality report to their consumers every year. You can often find them online or by calling your local water utility.

The EPA has a website to assist with finding your consumer confidence reports online,[7] but sometimes it's easier to make a phone call. Speaking with your water provider directly can offer additional insight you might not find in the official report. For example, you could ask them where they purchase the fluoride they add to the water supply and what type of fluoride is used. When my mom called her water supplier in Pennsylvania, she was told they temporarily stopped adding fluoride because of a shortage. When I called Seacoast Utility Authority in Palm Beach Gardens, the receptionist told me the local community (one of the wealthiest neighborhoods in South Florida) is ardent that fluoride not be added to the water supply.

Many water treatment personnel are well educated on fluoride and are personally and professionally against fluoridation. It is only natural to be suspicious when you see for yourself the skull and crossbones on the containers.[8] Water workers are the ones required to physically handle the chemicals, whether they agree with the practice or not.

If your water is fluoridated, you have two near term options for refusing force-fed fluoridation. One option is to drink bottled water verified to be low in fluoride. This was the course I pursued when I first suspected fluoride could be the cause of my acne. As with local

---

[6] Mahadevan, T.N., Meenaksy, V., Mishra, U.C., "Fluoride Cycling in Nature Through Precipitation." *Atmospheric Environmen,* vol. 20, issue 9, 1986, pp. 1745-1749.

[7] See "Find your local Consumer Confidence Report" (available at ofmpub.epa.gov/apex/safewater/f?p=136:102:).

[8] For a typical bag of fluoride added to water, see www.ProjectFree.Me/STOP.

water utilities, you can determine the fluoride content of various bottled water brands by researching their water quality reports online or you can contact the manufacturer directly. They should have this information readily available. Per FDA labeling requirements, if bottled water is labeled as de-ionized, purified, demineralized, or distilled, it will only contain fluoride in trace amounts unless fluoride is specifically listed as an added ingredient.[9]

Besides bottled water, the other option is to invest in a filter that removes fluoride from your regular water supply. Common carbon filters like Brita and Pur do not reduce fluoride, but reverse osmosis systems, de-ionizers, activated alumina, and distillation will remove most if not all fluoride from your drinking water. For more information on filters to remove fluoride, see ProjectFree.Me/Fluoride-Filters.

Fluoridated water is just the beginning, unfortunately. Now our story gets twistier. To simplify matters, here is a mnemonic device to help remember the five primary drinkable sources of fluoride exposure. You can count them on one hand as some of the most memorable characters from *Alice in Wonderland*. Our sordid cast of fluoridated potions includes Tweedledumb,[10] Tweedledee, the Red Queen, the White Rabbit and, of course, Johnny Depp.

If fluoridated water is Tweedledumb, then beverages made with fluoridated water are his equally contrariwise twin brother, Tweedledee. Soft drinks, juice, iced tea, coffee, and other beverages can all be made with fluoridated water, and if so they will contain fluoride in equal amounts or higher to the water with which they were produced.

Researchers at the University of Iowa measured fluoride concentrations of 332 soft drinks and found over 70 percent contained

---

[9] See "Bottled Water and Fluoridation" (available at www.cdc.gov/fluoridation/faqs/bottled_water.htm).

[10] Yep, the *b* is intentional.

fluoride at levels exceeding 0.6 ppm.[11] Researchers in New Zealand examined 532 juices and juice drinks and found fluoride levels ranging from .02 to 2.8 ppm.[12] The researchers in both studies accounted for the wide range of fluoride in large part because of variations in the amount of fluoride of the water used in production, proving Tweedledee right all along when he said, "If it was so, it might be; and if it were so, it would be; but as it isn't, it ain't. That's logic."

Beer falls in the Tweedledee category. If it is made from fluoridated water, it will contain fluoride. In 2002, researchers at King's College in London measured the fluoride content of various brands of beer, lager, and cider available in the United Kingdom.[13] They found a range of fluoride from .06 to .71 ppm and concluded that alcoholic beverages can be a significant source of fluoride even though they were not accounted for in the Total Diet Study when British officials estimated the average daily fluoride intake of its citizenry at 1.82 ppm.[14]

The British officials who conducted the fluoride portion of the Total Diet Study—two of whom hailed from the Ministry of Agriculture, two of whom hailed from the Laboratory of the Government Chemist, and one of whom was named Sherlock—did not suspect alcoholic beverages as a source of total dietary fluoride intake among British citizens and yet diligently accounted for fluoride in the tail meat of krill. Curiouser and curiouser, is it not?

If you don't have time to research the fluoride content of beer

---

[11] Hellman, J.R. et al., "Assessing fluoride levels of carbonated soft drinks." *Journal of the American Dental Association*, vol. 130, issue 11, Nov 1999, pp. 1593-1599.

[12] Kiritsy, M.C. et al., "Assessing fluoride concentrations of juices and juice-flavored drinks." *Journal of the American Dental Association*, vol. 127, issue 7, Jul 1996, pp. 895-902.

[13] Warnakulasuriya, Saman, "Fluoride content of alcoholic beverages," *Clinica Chimica Acta*, vol. 320, issues 1–2, Jun 2002, pp. 1–4.

[14] Walters, Charles B., Sherlock, John C., et al. "Dietary Intake of Fluoride in the United Kingdom and Fluoride Content of Some Foodstuffs," *Journal of the Science of Food and Agriculture*, vol. 34, issue 5, May 1983, pp. 523–528.

in advance, those brewed in continental Europe are generally a safe option since 97 percent of western Europe does not fluoridate its water supply.

Following Dumb and Dee is the Red Queen: wine. According to measurements from the 2005 USDA National Fluoride Database of Selected Foods and Beverages, wine contains an average fluoride content of 1.05 ppm for red wine and 2.02 ppm for white wine.[15] But these numbers tell us very little about the amount of fluoride contained in the bottle of wine on your kitchen counter. To understand that, it helps to know where the fluoride in wine comes from. Whereas beer is made from brewing certain grains in water, wine is made from crushing grapes. There's no water added.

The reason wine can contain significant amounts of fluoride is because of another Wonderland-esque character, the Western Grapeleaf Skeletonizer. A caterpillar exactly three inches tall with conspicuous tufts of long black poisonous spines, they feed on the undersides of grape leaves before transforming into luminescent blue-winged fairies (or moths).[16] The Omnivorous Leafroller, a bell-shaped character with a gray bat-like snout and brown ombre wings, is also to blame. To limit crop damage from Western Grapeleaf Skeletonizers and Omnivorous Leafrollers, some grape growers use a pesticide called cryolite which acts as a deadly poison in their grapeleaf-greedy bellies.

Cryolite was already featured in our story, just not by name. In the official version of the story of fluoridation outlined in chapter two, the young dentist hero's interest in fluoride was sparked when he realized it was the cause of the townspeople's brown teeth, a condition known as "Colorado Brown Stain." In Colorado Springs, where our hero settled, the community watershed was high in fluoride because it

---

[15] "USDA National Fluoride Database of Selected Beverages and Foods, Release 2," U.S. Department of Agriculture, Dec 2005.

[16] The University of California claims Western Grapeleaf Skeletonizers are only 0.6 inches in length but I defer to Lewis Caroll in all matters of caterpillar measurement.

contained deposits of cryolite from the rock formations of Pike's Peak. This is the same mineral, sodium hexafluoroaluminate, that is crushed and sold to grape growers under the trade name Kryocide, although now it is widely produced synthetically by combining sodium, fluoride, and aluminum.

Here's where your newfound insectology knowledge is put to good use. You see, Western Grapeleaf Skeletonizers and Omnivorous Leafrollers tend to confine their grapeleaf dining activities to California's Central Valley. To outsmart the Red Queen at her own game, all you need to do is choose wines from vineyards outside this region.

According to the California Department of Pesticide Regulation, the use of cryolite on wine grapes in 2013 was confined to four counties in Southern San Joaquin Valley: Fresno, Kings, Tulare, and Kern (plus one vineyard used by a large producer of inexpensive table wine in Yolo county).[17] Northern vineyards, including those in Napa and Sonoma, do not use cryolite. Neither do vineyards in southern or coastal areas like Temecula or Monterey.

To confirm, I wrote to every regional winery and growers association in California outside San Joaquin Valley and asked about their use of cryolite. The ones who replied either never heard of cryolite or verified they do not use it. I was also told that since cryolite is a fluoride product, some agricultural chemical companies like Wilbur Ellis won't sell it because of possible problems with residual fluoride in the groundwater.[18] On neighboring chessboards in Oregon and Washington states, vineyards are not treated with cryolite either.[19]

My skin verifies this information. I can drink reputable wine

---

[17] See "Pesticide Use Reporting—2013 Summary Data, 2013 County Summary Reports," California Department of Pesticide Regulation (available at www.cdpr.ca.gov/docs/pur/pur13rep/13_pur.htm).

[18] Personal email correspondence with Josie Gay, Executive Director, Heart of Sonoma Valley Winery Association, Oct 19, 2015.

[19] "No worries about cryolite here," *Seattle Times*, Jan 17, 2007.

from Sonoma, Columbia Valley, Europe, Argentina, New Zealand, and elsewhere without incident, but when I tried to politely sip a glass of California wine when visiting at a friend's home, my skin broke out before I left her house. Years later, I learned why. The winery is located in San Joaquin Valley.

In 1989, valiant challengers from abroad threatened the Red Queen's reign by limiting the fluoride content of all wine exported to Europe to 1 ppm. In response, Elf Atochem North America, the manufacturer of Kryocide, joined with other dark knights (i.e., Gowan Company, Gallo Winery, the Wine Institute, and California State University Fresno) to joust for an exception for California vineyards that use cryolite by raising their limit to 3 ppm[20]—an amount that is 50 percent higher than the Maximum Secondary Contaminant Level set by the EPA and over four times higher than the CDC's current recommendation for fluoridated water.[21] Their efforts were successful, and yet some California vineyards treated with cryolite still fail to meet the 3 ppm exception.[22]

The Red Queen monarchy extends to grape juice made from this region, as well. In a study of 43 ready-to-drink fruit juices, researchers from Tufts University measured the highest amount of fluoride in grape juice from Gerber at 6.8 ppm, well above the EPA's already inflated maximum contaminant level for fluoridated water of 4 ppm.[23] Even fruit juices and other fruit drinks that don't have the word "grape" in their name often contain blends of grape juice with significant amounts of fluoride.

---

[20] "Kryocide Advisory on Use of Cryolite to Control Insects on Grapes," Elf Atochem North America, Inc. (available at www.fluoridealert.org/content/kryocide-advisory-grapes/).

[21] See "Review of Fluoride Drinking Water Standard" (available at http://water.epa.gov/drink/contaminants/basicinformation/fluoride.cfm#four).

[22] "Kryocide Advisory," Elf Atochem (available at www.fluoridealert.org/content/kryocide-advisory-grapes/).

[23] Stannard, Jan G., et al. "Fluoride levels and fluoride contamination of fruit juices," *The Journal of Clinical Pediatric Dentistry*, vol. 16, issue 1, 1991, pp. 38-40.

In 2002, a cryolite supplier petitioned the National Organic Standards Board to have it included on the list of allowed pesticides for organic production.[24] You can tell the petition was proofread by dentists because of phrases like "as a mineral, the only residues remaining are basic elements found in nature," and also because of the A+ cartoon tooth sticker at the top of the page. Despite this strong argument, the petition was rejected and as a result, organic fruit juices contain the least amount of fluoride since the use of cryolite is prohibited on organic crops.[25]

But don't forget about Tweedledee and his propensity to confuse matters. If juice is made with fluoridated water it can still contain fluoride even if it is labeled as organic. "If it was so, it might be." Got it?

The next character in our lineup is the White Rabbit. If you follow him deep enough down the rabbit hole, he will eventually reveal the whole matrix. He first hops across the page when Alice chases him into Wonderland, the same way researchers chase dairy down the rabbit hole of dietary causes for acne.

In 2005, a study headed by a nutritional epidemiologist from Harvard School of Public Health analyzed questionnaires from 47,355 teenage females from the famous Nurse's Health Study and found a positive correlation between acne and dairy consumption, particularly skim milk.[26] His team published follow-up studies in 2006[27] and

---

[24] Formella, Timothy M., "Petition for the listing of Cryolite on the USDA National List of Allowed and Prohibited Substances," Cerexagri, Inc., submitted to National Organic Standards Board, Washington, D.C., Oct 25, 2002.

[25] For information on the history of substances, including cryolite, petitioned for inclusion on the National Organics Standards list see www.ams.usda.gov/rules-regulations/organic/national-list/co.

[26] Adebamowo, C.A., et al. "High school dietary dairy intake and teenage acne." *Journal of the American Academy of Dermatology,* vol. 52, issue 2, Feb 2005, pp. 207-214.

[27] Adebamowo, C.A., et al., "Milk consumption and acne in adolescent girls," *Dermatology Online Journal,* vol. 12, 2006, p. 1.

2008,[28] both of which supported the correlation between milk consumption—especially skim milk—and adolescent acne.

Dermatologists were confused by these results. If milk causes acne in adolescents, surely it must have something to do with the hormones milk contains. In his response to the Harvard study published in the same journal issue, dermatologist Guy *"Sassypants"* Webster begins, "Diet causes acne. [*snap*] No it does not!"[29] He then argues that the study's findings "seem to exonerate bovine hormones as the acne factor in milk because they would presumably be mostly in the lipid fractions."[30] In other words, whole milk should cause more acne than skim milk because of its higher fat content, and thus its higher hormone content; therefore, diet is not the cause of acne; therefore, drugs are the only solution. But that does not appear to be what is happening in the wonderland of acne research.

To understand what is going on with milk and acne, it helps to ponder a question posed to Alice at a certain tea party you might remember her attending, uninvited. "Why is a raven like a writing desk?" Excellent question, don't you think? It leads one to wonder what makes one thing one thing and another thing the other thing save someone says it's so? Why is milk milk and not a raven or a writing desk?

If you ask the U.S. Food and Drug Administration, the answer is very clear. According to the U.S. Code of Federal Regulations Title 21, Section 131, Subpart B, milk is "the lacteal secretion, practically free from colostrum, obtained by the complete milking of one or more healthy cows."[31] It is unclear what the resulting liquid is called

---

28 Adebamowo, C.A. et al., "Milk consumption and acne in teenaged boys," *Journal of the American Academy of Dermatology*, vol. 58, 2008, pp. 787-793.

29 Sass in italics added for emphasis.

30 Webster, G. F., "Commentary: diet and acne," *Journal of the American Academy of Dermatology*, vol. 58, 2008, pp. 794–795.

31 U.S. Food and Drug Administration. "Title 21—Food and Drugs; Section 131—Milk and Cream," U.S. Government Printing Office, April 1, 1999.

following an incomplete milking of a goat who is feeling a little under the weather, for example, but their definition sounds reasonable enough so far.

The guidelines go on to explain that milk "shall contain not less than 8 1/4 percent milk solids not fat and not less than 3 1/4 percent milkfat." That seems unnecessarily demanding of both God and Mother Nature, but okay. They continue, "Milk may have been adjusted by separating part of the milkfat therefrom, or by adding thereto cream, concentrated milk, dry whole milk, skim milk, concentrated skim milk, or nonfat dry milk." In Section 133, Subpart A, under the definition of milk used for cheese, they add, "Water, in a sufficient quantity to reconstitute concentrated and dry forms, may be added."[32]

To quote the headline from Emily Green's article in the *Los Angeles Times*, "Is milk still milk?"[33] If you ask Wikipedia, your grandmother, a suckling baby, or even the FDA-equivalent in another country, the definition of milk you receive will likely be a little different, and probably a lot simpler. According to Wikipedia, "Milk is a white liquid produced by the mammary glands of mammals."[34] The end. As you can see, the FDA definition stretches this concept of milk much further.

Virtually all words—milk, raven, writing desk, Real Kraft Cheese—are brimming with this kind of existential wiggle-room that shrewd food manufacturers use to their advantage. Humpty Dumpty elucidates this point quite eloquently when he tells Alice, "When I use a word, it means just what I choose it to mean—no more, no less... I can manage the whole lot of them! Impenetrability!"

What if the teenagers in the Harvard study weren't drinking

---

[32] U.S. Food and Drug Administration. "Title 21—Food and Drugs; Section 133—Cheeses and Related Cheese Products" U.S. Government Printing Office, April 1, 1999.

[33] Green, Emily. "Is Milk Still Milk," *Los Angeles Times*, Aug 2, 2000.

[34] https://en.wikipedia.org/wiki/milk

milk at all, like that guy in *The Matrix* who sold out Neo for a digital steak? What if they only *thought* they were drinking milk but it was really an imposter made of the same stuff as chocolate-chip-*"flavored"* cookies or *"bac'n"* bits or powdered country *"lemonade."*[35]

In her article for the *LA Times*, Emily Green describes the frankenstein process industrialized milk goes through to be recreated after leaving the utter.[36] First, it is shipped to a processing plant where centrifuges are used to separate it into fat, protein, and various other solids and liquids. Once segregated, they are then reconstituted to standardized levels for whole, low-fat, and skim milks. "Whole" milk is the closest to original cow's milk, but it's still not the same thing, and it's certainly not whole. When skim milk is first produced it is a watery, chalky, blue-tinged shadow of real milk's natural self, which is why some people still refer to it as "Blue John." As one traditional dairy farmer put it, the product in the grocery store we commonly think of as milk is no longer milk, but rather it is a reconstituted milk-flavored beverage.

According to the USDA National Fluoride Database of Selected Beverages and Foods, skim milk has a mean fluoride concentration of 0.03 ppm.[37] So does milk with 1 or 2 percent milkfat. But mean averages don't mean much in Wonderland where there are only four branches of Arithmetic: Ambition, Distraction, Uglification, and Derision. As the Red Queen has already demonstrated, government measurements of the fluoride content of various foods are meant to be more of a nonsensical guideline than a respectable gauge of the amount of fluoride contained in the product you just purchased at the grocery store.

To make skim milk palatable and more acceptable aesthetically,

---

[35] For more fake foods, see "19 Foods that Aren't Foods" by Mandy Oaklander, *Prevention*, Jul 1, 2013.

[36] Green, "Milk," *LA Times*, 2000.

[37] "USDA National Fluoride Database of Selected Beverages and Foods, Release 2," U.S. Department of Agriculture, Dec 2005.

manufacturers add powdered milk solids. Could powdered milk solids—not hormones—be the reason industrialized skim milk-flavored beverages are correlated with acne? Researchers tend to go on and on about dairy as if ravens and writing desks have *so much* in common, but the studies on powdered milk solids are scant and studies on the fluoride content of powdered milk solids are even scanter. Let's see if we can find some clues.

In the original Harvard study, other dairy products found to have a positive correlation with acne were cottage cheese, cream cheese, instant breakfast drinks, and sherbet. Each of these products is commonly made from skim milk or contains milk protein concentrates. (You don't even want to know what kind of dairy goes into what the FDA classifies as sherbet.[38]) In the USDA fluoride database, milk solids are not listed, but powdered cream substitute is noted as having a mean fluoride concentration of 1.12 ppm. In a 1952 article entitled "A Survey of the Literature of Dental Caries," the authors reference a study conducted ten years prior (before fluoridation) when researchers found the fluorine content of cow milk solids to vary from 0.4 to 4.4 ppm.[39]

---

[38] Fine, don't listen to me. Here it is: "(b) Optional dairy ingredients. The optional dairy ingredients referred to in paragraph (a) of this section are: Cream, dried cream, plastic cream (sometimes known as concentrated milkfat), butter, butter oil, milk, concentrated milk, evaporated milk, superheated condensed milk, sweetened condensed milk, dried milk, skim milk, concentrated skim milk, evaporated skim milk, condensed skim milk, sweetened condensed skim milk, sweetened condensed part-skim milk, nonfat dry milk, sweet cream buttermilk, condensed sweet cream buttermilk, dried sweet cream buttermilk, skim milk that has been concentrated and from which part of the lactose has been removed by crystallization, and whey and those modified whey products (e.g., reduced lactose whey, reduced minerals whey, and whey protein concentrate) that have been determined by FDA to be generally recognized as safe (GRAS) for use in this type of food. Water may be added, or water may be evaporated from the mix. The sweet cream buttermilk and the concentrated sweet cream buttermilk or dried sweet cream buttermilk, when adjusted with water to a total solids content of 8.5 percent, has a titratable acidity of not more than 0.17 percent calculated as lactic acid. The term "milk" as used in this section means cow's milk." SOURCE: U.S. Food and Drug Administration. "Title 21—Food and Drugs; Section 135—Frozen Desserts" U.S. Government Printing Office, April 1, 1999.

[39] Jeans, P.C. chairman, "A Survey of the Literature of Dental Caries," National Research Council, 1952, p. 356.

So how much fluoride is commonly contained in milk solids? I'm not sure anyone knows. In a 2012 study published in the *British Journal of Nutrition*, researchers in Iran found high levels of fluoride in certain powdered milk formulas and concluded they were likely caused by water used in the factory during the production process.[40] Skim milk solids are widely manufactured through a technique called spray drying.[41] In this technique, the milk is processed as a slurry in a rotating cylinder before being dehydrated. The Iranian researchers postulate that when the water from the slurry vaporizes, fluoride remains concentrated in the finished product. If their theory is correct, milk solids processed in plants with fluoridated water would contain higher amounts of fluoride than other milk solids.

We are deep in the rabbit hole now and I can't say with certainty if we will reach the other side, but how funny it would seem to come out among the people who walk with their heads downwards. It is possible dairy products correlate with acne for reasons other than the fluoride content of milk solids, or perhaps they do not correlate at all. My skin cannot attest to the fluoride content of industrialized milk products because I have not consumed them since discovering my fluoroderma.[42] I still drink milk and eat plenty of cottage cheese, yogurt, and other dairy products daily, but they are not the morphed variety found only in Wonderland.

Instead of purchasing milk-like beverages at the grocery story, the majority of my dairy products are now delivered fresh from a traditional farm (i.e., where cows live on pastures) just like when my grandfather was a milkman in the '40s and '50s before the industrial needs of World War II fully reshaped the American diet—and before

---

[40] Mohave, Amir Hossein, "Determination of fluoride concentration in powdered milk in Iran 2010," *British Journal of Nutrition*, vol. 107, 2012, pp. 1077–1079.

[41] https://en.wikipedia.org/wiki/Spray_drying

[42] You might be wondering why I don't just drink some skim milk and see what happens—you know, in the name of science. Truth is, I made the mistake of reading *Skinny Bitch* several years ago and now I can never drink grocery store milk again. Ever. Thanks, bitches.

acne was an accepted part of everyday life. If you decide it is time to wakeup from Wonderland altogether, you can learn more about how to locate a dairy farmer near you by visiting ProjectFree.Me/Food-Supply.

The final character in our drinkable lineup is the colorful, lovable, mad-as-a-hatter Hatter. After failing to impress the Queen of Hearts with his rendition of "Twinkle, Twinkle, Little Bat," the Hatter is sentenced to death for "murdering the time." He escapes but time is unforgiving and halts the Hatter at 6 o'clock in the evening, leaving him in a perpetual tea party, a Victorian version of Margaritaville.

Studying the topic of fluoride and tea is enough to drive one mad. Remember that statistic dentists like to quote about how fluoride is the thirteenth most abundant natural element in the earth's crust? Tea plants happen to be the only edible plants that uptake natural fluoride from the soil in large amounts, so of course that's the one we decide to build our empires around.[43] The amount of fluoride in a single cup of tea varies widely. Most studies report levels from 1 to 5 ppm depending on the age of the plant, the chemical characteristics of the growing region, and the length of steeping time.[44]

In 2010, researchers from the Medical College of Georgia discovered the fluoride content of tea is even higher than previously thought.[45] Four patients were each diagnosed with skeletal fluorosis because of their advanced joint pain and excessive tea consumption (FYI, one will only be diagnosed with skeletal fluorosis if one's symptoms are advanced and one's fluoride consumption excessive).[46]

---

[43] See: Rose, Sarah, *For All the Tea in China: How England Stole the World's Favorite Drink and Changed History.* New York: Penguin Books, 2011.

[44] Ruan, J.Y.; Wong, M.H., "Accumulation of Fluoride and aluminum related to different varieties of tea plants," *Environmental Geochemistry and Health*, vol. 23, issue 1, Mar 2001, pp. 53-63.

[45] Public release from the Medical College of Georgia, "Tea Contains More Fluoride Than Once Thought," Georgia Regents University, July 14, 2010.

[46] For more studies regarding tea consumption and skeletal fluorosis, see fluoridealert.org/studies/tea03/.

When researchers measured the amount of fluoride in the brands of tea the patients were drinking, however, they were puzzled to find the concentrations were very low. Where was the fluoride that was causing their skeletal fluorosis?

Realizing that tea also absorbs inordinate amounts of aluminum, the researchers wondered if the aluminum was somehow hiding the fluoride. They performed an experiment to test their hypothesis by dissolving the insoluble aluminum fluoride bonds found in tea prior to measuring for fluoride. Their results showed that fluoride concentrations in seven common store-bought brands of black tea were up to *three hundred percent higher* than previous measurements indicated.

To be clear, the type of tea we are discussing here is tea from the camellia sinensis plant. It commonly comes in black, green, and white varieties with white being the lowest in fluoride since the leaves are picked when young. Ceylon, pekoe, oolong, pu-erh, Darjeeling, earl grey, instant—these are all ways of referring to tea from the camellia sinensis plant and thus are susceptible to fluoride accumulation.

Some sources claim organic tea is lower in fluoride, but I have not found any information to confirm that assertion. Some high quality matcha tea from Japan is said to be low in fluoride, as well. In theory tea plants grown without soil, i.e., hydroponically, could be cultivated to have low levels of fluoride, but I do not know of any that are commercially available.[47] Truthfully, I have not looked very hard because I already switched to herbal tea by the time I realized my acne was caused by fluoride.

Herbal tea is another raven/writing desk situation. Technically,

---

[47] In a 2013 article by Chinese researchers studying the fluoride content of hydroponically grown tea plants, they found the aroma of the tea leaves decreased as the fluoride content increased, leading them to conclude that "elevated concentrations of [fluoride] during growth have negative effects on the aroma and flavor quality of tea leaves." SOURCE: Li, Chunlei, et al. "Effect of fluoride on aroma of tea leaves," *Fluoride*, vol. 46, issue 1, Jan-Mar 2013, pp. 25-28.

it's an infusion, or tisane, which is defined simply as a drink prepared by soaking the leaves of a plant in liquid. This description would seem to apply to tea as well but tea experts assure us it does not. Tea is tea and tisanes are not tea. If enough of us nod in unison then it will be declared so, as is the case with all language. Tea that is not tea includes peppermint, chamomile, dandelion, and many other flavorful varieties. I find the taste of raspberry leaf is a nice substitute if you are craving traditional black tea. If you drink tea for an energy boost, my sensei, Tim Ferris, recommends yerba mate.

So there you have it. The five common drinkable sources of suspected fluoride exposure are fluoridated water (Tweedledumb), beverages made with fluoridated water (Tweedledee), wine from the Fresno region of California (the Red Queen), frankenmilk (the White Rabbit), and tea (the Mad Hatter). But before we move on to the next scene, there is more we can learn about fluoride from the experience of hatters.

Prior to the mid 1900s, hatters were a mainstay of society for centuries. Someone had to create all the fashionable hats everyone thought they were required to wear while out in public. Hats were made from the pelts of small animals which the hatters turned into felt by removing the fur from the skin. Respectable hat manufacturers claimed to use camel urine to break down the necessary chemical bonds in the pelts. Unfortunately for hatters and hat-wearers, camels aren't the thirstiest of creatures and sometimes camel urine was hard to come by in places like France and England. When faced with camel urine shortages, resourceful hatters used their own instead.[48]

Over time, French hatters made a curious observation. If a hatter happened to have syphilis and happened to be taking mercury chloride as a treatment for the disease, his urine was especially effective at making felt. How fortuitous.

---

[48] Kitzmiller , Kathryn J., "The Not-So-Mad Hatter: Occupational Hazards of Mercury," Science Connections, Chemical Abstracts Service, a division of the American Chemical Society (available at www.cas.org/news/insights/science-connections/mad-hatter).

Hatters started using mercury, a known neurotoxin, for felting and soon afterwards phrases like "mad as a hatter" came into common usage. Symptoms of mercurial poisoning were prevalent amongst hatters and included insomnia, depression, loose teeth, digestive problems, shaking so severe it inhibited basic functions like walking and speaking, paranoia, mental instability, miscarriage, hallucination, and early death.[49]

In 1860, a physician in New Jersey named J. Addison Freeman published an article entitled "Mercurial Disease Among Hatters" which outlined the illness and recommended steps for prevention which were promptly ignored by the American hatmaking industry and government regulators.[50] In 1878, an inspection of 25 hat companies in Newark found that a quarter of the 1,589 hatters exhibited mercurial disease.[51] By the turn of the century, both France and Great Britain passed legislation to protect hatters from mercury poisoning making the condition rare in those countries, but American hatters continued going mad for decades.

By 1934, the U.S. Public Health Service estimated that 80 percent of American felt workers, most of whom were poor immigrants, suffered from mercurial tremors. Yet the practice did not end until *nine years later* when hat manufacturers volunteered to use hydrogen peroxide, a readily available substitute, since mercury supplies were needed to produce detonators for World War II.[52]

There are a number of lessons from our mad hatter history we

---

[49] Clark, Claudia. *Radium Girls, Women, and Industrial Health Reform: 1910-1935,* The University of North Carolina Press, Chapel Hill and London, 1997.

[50] Freeman, J. Addison, "Mercurial Disease Among Hatters". *Transactions of the Medical Society of New Jersey,* 1860, pp. 61-64 (as cited at "Mad hatter disease," on Wikipedia.

[51] Dennis, L, "Hatting: As effecting the health of operatives". Report of the New Jersey State Board of Health 2, 1878, pp. 67–85 (as cited in Wedeen, R.P., "Were the hatters of New Jersey 'mad'?" *American Journal of Industrial Medicine,* vol. 16, issue 2, 1989, pp. 225–233).

[52] Wedeen, R.P., "Were the hatters of New Jersey 'mad'?" *American Journal of Industrial Medicine,* vol. 16, issue 2, 1989, pp. 225–233.

can apply to our current experience with fluoride. First, just because an expert at the top of his profession thinks something is a good idea, it does not mean it is safe for humans. He might turn out to be a crazy French hatter with syphilis (or a dentist).

Second, as with fluoride, mercury is a natural element that occurs naturally in the earth's natural crust, ranking just behind silver in natural abundance. Clearly, just because an element is natural does not mean it is safe for humans.

Third, it took the United States government over eighty years after the publication of Freeman's article on mercurial disease among hatters (plus a *little* extra incentive from WWII) to end the use of mercury in the hatmaking industry, showing that just because a practice has been in widespread use for decades *does not mean it is safe for humans.* When we decide to do something dumb, sometimes we keep on doing it for a very long time. (You know this.)

Finally, in his account of mad hatters syndrome in New Jersey, Richard Wedeen notes the most remarkable aspect of the hatters' story is that they expressed no anger about their working conditions. The minutes from their association meetings make no reference to any of the symptoms of mercurial poisoning. The medical community, the government, the general public, and the hatters themselves all seemed thoroughly unconcerned by the raging lunacy exhibited by the people creating their pretty hats. So is the case with fluoride.

As the wise Cheshire Cat explained to young Alice, everyone is mad in Wonderland. It's to be expected.

Tweedledumb and Tweedledee
Fetch only plain tap water.
Fresno's Queen, White Rabbit scheme,
Mad Hatter's tea is hotter.

*****

The "EAT ME" Cakes

I have to admit, the *Alice in Wonderland* theme seemed like a fun and fitting analogy but now that I'm digging into it, I'm starting to wonder something. Hear me out. There are all kinds of theories about Lewis Carroll incorporating adult sexual themes or drugs, etcetera into his famous children's books (you write about *one* caterpillar smoking a hookah on a magic mushroom...), but all the references to fluoride are starting to seem a little more than coincidental, you know what I mean?

Take Alice's encounter with Humpty Dumpty, for example. She meets him sitting there on top of the wall and you know exactly where that chapter is going. None of the king's horses or even his men could put Humpty back together. If you repeat the words of the nursery rhyme and then close your eyes and picture Humpty Dumpty, what do you see? An egg? Wrong! Humpty Dumpty was a cannon. It was used in Colchester, England in 1648 during the English Civil War until an opposing cannon knocked down the wall beneath it, causing Humpty to fall to the ground never to be recovered.[53] Go ahead and repeat the nursery rhyme again. See? No egg.[54] Lewis Carroll is the one who is credited with turning Humpty Dumpty into a story about broken eggshells. And guess what's high in fluoride. Yep. Eggshells.

As with humans, birds bioaccumulate fluoride. In an article published in the *Journal of Wildlife Diseases*, researchers in Norway measured fluoride concentrations in 405 wild herring eggs and discovered that eggs found near aluminum smelters were significantly

---

[53] At least that's what it says at knowledgenuts.com.

[54] "Humpty Dumpty sat on a wall. Humpty Dumpty had a great fall. All the king's horses and all the king's men couldn't put Humpty together again." See? Still no egg. But it does leave one wondering why they named their cannon Humpty.

higher in fluoride.[55] They also measured for fluoride in 42 herring femur bones and found a positive correlation between the amount of fluoride in a bird's femur bone and in the shells the bird produced. Researchers in Poland performed similar tests on domestic hens. The bones from chickens who drank fluoridated water were significantly higher in fluoride than the bones of chickens in a control group.[56]

Why should you care if the chickens you eat are bioaccumulating fluoride? Most people don't eat eggshells or chicken bones, right? Wrong again! (What's up with you today?) Most people do eat chicken bones, and they are consuming *outrageous* amounts of fluoride at the same time.

Chicken caused my absolute worst acne flareups. Soon after diagnosing my fluoroderma, my husband and I decided to move to a neighboring county that is unfluoridated. I was excited about simple things like being able to take baths again and order soup at a restaurant. While we were still house hunting, I made the mistake of ordering wonton soup from a local Chinese take-out place. Within hours, my face was Freddy Krueger. I called the water company who verified the water was unfluoridated, and then I called the restaurant to ask about the soup. They proudly explained it was made in the traditional manner by simmering a chicken carcass for several hours to make a mineral-rich broth. Ah-ha! That explained it. I was basically eating dissolved chicken bones.

I had a similar experience after accidentally purchasing chicken hot dogs instead of the regular beef version I usually bought. It was a high quality brand made from "all natural" chicken raised without antibiotics or artificial hormones, but none of that mattered.

Chicken hot dogs and other chicken products are often made

---

[55] Vikoren, T., and G. Stuve. "Fluoride Exposure and Selected Characteristics of Eggs and Bones of the Herring Gull (Larus Argentatus) and the Common Gull (Larus Canus)." *Journal of Wildlife Diseases,* vol. 32, issue 2, 1996, p. 190.

[56] Machaliński B. "Concentration and distribution of fluorine in hen's eggs as an aspect of selected biological parameters," *Annales Academiae Medicae Stetinensis,* vol. 42, 1996, pp. 25-38.

from an industrialized product referred to in the food industry as mechanically-deboned meat (MDM). I don't know about you, but when I think of the term "mechanically-deboned meat," I picture a fancy laser gizmo cutting meat from the bone with machine-like precision. But Wikipedia describes mechanically-deboned meat as a paste-like meat product made from forcing pureed chicken under high pressure through a sieve or similar device to separate the bone from the edible meat tissue.[57] Oh.

When this process is used to create chicken products, the fluoride content can be astronomically high due to residue from chicken bones and other high fluoride bits that end up in the finished product. In a study published in the *Journal of Agricultural and Food Chemistry*, researchers from Oregon State University measured the fluoride content of various foods made with mechanically separated poultry.[58] They found pureed infant foods were highest in fluoride, up to 8.63 ppm, and that a single serving could contain 87 percent of the upper "safe" limit for fluoride for a six month old infant (parents beware). Chicken sticks were the next highest, up to 6 ppm, with a single serving providing over half a milligram of fluoride.

The other two poultry categories they measured, canned meats and luncheon meats, were also high in fluoride with values as high as 3.65 ppm. Turkey products contain less fluoride than chicken products but only because the bones are firmer and less likely to end up in the meat. When the researchers measured turkey bones directly, they were found to contain more fluoride than the chicken bones contained, something to keep in mind if you plan on making soup from your Thanksgiving leftovers.

Here is an even dirtier secret dentists will never tell you. Fluoridated drinking water is not the primary reason chicken parts are

---

[57] See https://en.wikipedia.org/wiki/Mechanically_separated_meat.

[58] Fein, Noelle J., Cerklewski, Florian L., "Fluoride Content of Foods Made with Mechanically Separated Chicken," *Journal of Agricultural and Food Chemistry,* vol. 49, issue 9, 2001, pp.4284-4286.

high in fluoride. Humpty Dumpty had a great fall, indeed.

As we learned in our discussion of California wine, the food and beverage industry (unlike the medical community) has figured out that fluoride is very good at being toxic. According to an EPA ruling from July 15, 2005, the legal limit for fluoride pesticide residue on animal feed is 130 ppm.[59] *One hundred and thirty*. The CDC recommendation for fluoridated drinking water is only 0.7 ppm. The EPA does not have a tolerance for fluoride residue in animal products because they determined "there is no reasonable expectation of finite residues in livestock."[60] It appears the EPA does not know where chicken soup comes from or how to look up chicken research on PubMed.

Regardless, can you imagine what chicken feed with up to 130 ppm fluoride is doing to their little chicken thyroids and bird-sized pineal glands? Is it absurd to think about chicken thyroids and pineal glands? I think it's absurd not to, but that's just me. What do you think?[61]

The studies I've found on the bioaccumulation of fluoride in chickens are focused on chicken bones or mechanically separated meat, but as we've seen with other studies, fluoride can accumulate in tissues other than bone. I've found that my skin does not react to commercially-raised chicken breast as long as it is not cooked on the bone, but bone-in chicken, chicken skin, or even a small bite with

---

[59] "Sulfuryl fluoride: Pesticide Tolerance." Federal Register, vol. 70, issue 135, Jul 2005, pp. 40899-40908.

[60] "Cryolite Summary Document Registration Review: Initial Docket March 2011," Environmental Protection Agency, Mar 16, 2011.

[61] "...the pineal gland in birds is located under the skull in the middle of the bird's forehead. The skull in this area is actually thin enough for light to penetrate through the skin and skull bone to directly stimulate the pineal gland, which also has photoreceptors. It is like a third eye. So even a chicken that is blind can still "see the light" and continue to have a relatively normal reproductive system as long as they have the right exposure to light and dark periods." From "The Avian Pineal Gland: Even a Blind Chicken Can See Spring Coming" by Elsbeth Upton at *Backyard Poultry* (available at www.backyardpoultrymag.com/the-avian-pineal-gland-even-a-blind-chicken-can-see-spring-coming/).

gristle will cause a fluoroderma reaction if the chicken was not raised to strict organic standards.

I experimented with making chicken soup from a large national brand of organic chicken purchased at the grocery store but my skin still had a reaction. I suspect either the chicken was provided fluoridated water or perhaps there is some leeway in the organic certification process. I gave up on chicken soup for a few years but then one Thanksgiving, we purchased a beautiful organic heritage turkey from our local farmer. I couldn't throw out the carcass without first turning it into soup. It made a thick golden broth that gelled like jello when it cooled and did not cause a single breakout on my skin.

Now I eat grilled chicken legs regularly, crispy skin and all, and I consume more chicken soup than Jack Canfield's soul. The key is to purchase organic chicken products from a farm you trust. Chicken labeled natural or free-range is not the same as organic. It might still be low in fluoride if the chicken did not consume feed sprayed with fluoride-based pesticides, but you would need to ask the farmer to verify. The organic certification is expensive for small farmers who sometimes raise their chickens to organic standards but can't afford the label. I purchase chicken from the same farmer I found for milk. For more information on how to find a traditional farmer near you, see ProjectFree.Me/Food-Supply.

I know from personal experience it can be a difficult adjustment to start buying organic chicken instead of the cheaper factory-farmed variety. But once I made the switch, I never once regretted it. I love supporting my local farmer, having clear skin, and also I'm just a sucker for those little chicken faces.

If Humpty Dumpty did not convince you as to Lewis Carroll's anti-fluoride subtext in *Alice in Wonderland*, let's talk about the Walrus and the Carpenter for a moment, shall we? What jumps out at you when you think about walruses? It's those two ridiculously long canine teeth that protrude from their upper jaw like elephant tusks, right? You're not going to believe this, but they contain fluoride.[62]

Like birds and humans, marine species bioaccumulate fluoride in their teeth and bones. Researchers have found that the fluoride content of salt water seems to increase with its salinity,[63] but it also becomes less bioavailable because of the increased mineral content of water with higher salinity.[64] Fluoride in salt water has a different structure than fluoride in fresh water because of sea water's high magnesium content. Approximately half of the fluoride in sea water is bound with magnesium.[65]

(FYI, swimming in the ocean does not have a negative effect on my skin, although when my fluoroderma was at its worst in Delray Beach I remember developing a stinging rash if I shaved my legs within a few hours of going into the ocean. That rarely happens to me anymore.)

While most of us don't eat walrus tusks, some foods do contain fish bones that are high in fluoride. For example, canned salmon often comes packed with the skin and bones. Sardines and anchovies are commonly served whole. The fluoride in seafood is a mystery I have not yet been able to completely figure out. Some sources claim it is caused by environmental pollution, both natural and industrial, while other sources claim all seafood, even protein from fish, is naturally high in fluoride. My skin does not break out from things like fish, shellfish, sea salt, or even seafood bisque which is prepared by simmering seafood shells in water to make a stock.

At one point I thought perhaps the fluoride in fish bones might not provoke my acne, but I tested this theory to the extreme on a trip

---

[62] "A Survey of the Literature of Dental Caries," National Academy of Sciences, National Research Council, U.S. Committee on Dental Health, Washington D.C., Oct 13, 1952, p. 332.

[63] Weinstein, Leonard H, Davison, A., *Fluorides in the Environment: Effects on Plants and Animals*, CABI Publishing, Cambridge, MA, p. 11.

[64] Camargo, Julio A., "Fluoride toxicity to aquatic organisms: a review," *Chemosphere*, vol. 50, issue 3, Jan 2003, pp. 251-264.

[65] *Ibid.*, p. 11.

to Italy where we dined on the Mediterranean coast at a restaurant with an entire page on the menu devoted to anchovy appetizers. The waiter convinced me to order the "anchovy fantasy platter" to taste a few of their most popular dishes. He brought out a plate of six whole anchovies, perfectly grilled, caught fresh that morning. Then he brought a plate of fried anchovies. Then stuffed. Then marinated. Then things got a little fuzzy, but I know there were more anchovies involved. It was clear by the next morning that anchovies can cause fluoroderma, at least when eaten to excess.

We'll talk more about seafood in chapter six. For now, just know that avoiding fish bones will help reduce your fluoride exposure. Sorry to break the bad news to all you fish bone lovers out there!

Now about that Carpenter. Carpenters work with the natural grain of wood to transform raw plant parts into finished products that become part of our everyday lives. Isn't it obvious? Carroll is hinting about breakfast cereal there, *duh*. (Get it? Transforming plant parts into stuff we use daily? Nevermind.) Grains on their own don't contain significant amounts of fluoride, but extruded breakfast cereals like *"puffed"* rice, *"flaked"* corn, and *"shredded"* wheat often do. The reason is because they are processed with the same type of technique used in the manufacturing of milk solids.

In the production of most commercial breakfast cereals, grains (usually rice, oats, corn, or wheat) are mixed with water, processed into a slurry, and then placed in a machine called an extruder where they are forced through a small hole at a high temperature and pressure, shaping them into lucky stars or whatever shape the mascot on the box dictates. When the water from the slurry evaporates, any fluoride it contained is left concentrated in the cereal. One study of cereals processed in fluoridated versus non-fluoridated regions found significant differences in their fluoride content, with cereals processed in fluoridated water ranging from 3.8 to 6.3 ppm.[66]

Virtually all boxed breakfast cereals are manufactured with this extrusion process, even "organic" ones found in the health food store. Since the fluoride in water is not a pesticide, it does not count for organic labelling purposes.

You can still eat cereal for breakfast if you have fluoroderma, but the best option is the old fashioned method of purchasing fresh whole grains and making them yourself. Preparing whole oats might be a little more cumbersome than pouring yourself a bowl of kibble for breakfast, but it's really not that difficult, especially if you set the oats out the night before to soak in an acidic medium (such as water with a spoonful of yogurt, whey, or apple cider vinegar). This was the tradition prior to boxed breakfast cereals coming into fashion and is basically the first step in fermentation, a longstanding traditional process that makes grains and other foods more nutritious and easier to digest.

Oats are just one option. If you've been letting cartoon tigers influence your breakfast decisions, you might be pleasantly surprised by the variety of *real* cereals you've been missing out on. Quinoa, millet, buckwheat, amaranth—these are all just as easy to prepare as oats. But for me, I generally skip breakfast cereal most days. Instead, I like to eat eggs from the farm with bright yolks the color of orange sunshine. If you use a cast iron skillet, you don't even need to wash the pan.

Okay, so the Carpenter and the cereal connection was a stretch. Clearly we're just riding out this *Alice in Wonderland* theme because a) it's fun and b) it's a proven medical fact that anti-fluoridationists like a good conspiracy theory. While we're at it, we might as well introduce our own character that Lewis Carroll would have included in Wonderland if he really were writing about fluoride.

---

[66] Warren, J.J., Levy, S.M. "Current and future role of fluoride in nutrition." *Dental Clinics of North America*, vol. 42, 2003, pp. 225-243 (as cited at fluoridealert.org/content/processed-drinks/).

As you recall, Tweedledumb represents fluoridated water. Tweedledee represents beverages made with fluoridated water. Tweedledodo, the younger brother of Dumb and Dee, represents *food* made with fluoridated water.

Foods that absorb fluoridated water during the cooking process will add to the fluoride load on your skin. Pasta, rice, mashed potatoes, steamed vegetables—these are all potential sources of fluoride because of the water they contain. Think of Tweedledodo as "that guy" who worms his way into a place at your table when you run into him while you're eating out with your friends. For some reason I always picture him wearing a t-shirt with a big F on it and a beanie with a propellor on top, but of course he's not that obvious about it. Most menus include enough grilled, roasted, or sautéed foods that it is possible to avoid making room for him at your table without looking rude. He tends to have an aversion to salads, too. (Typical guy.)[67]

There is one major food source of fluoride that we still need to add to our list. I know we are supposed to have dropped the Wonderland theme by now, but this one is just too weird. Remember the "EAT ME" cake Alice consumed when she needed a way to grow taller so she could reach the golden key for the door leading from the bottom of the rabbit hole into the Wonderland garden? As Carroll describes, it was a little cake "on which the words 'EAT ME' were beautifully marked in currants." Because I lived in Scotland, I know this one: currants is the British code word for *raisins*. (You should let that one sink in for a moment.)

Raisins are high in fluoride for the same reason some wine is high in fluoride. Virtually all raisins in the United States are grown in the central San Joaquin Valley or, as Western Grapeleaf Skeletonizers and Omnivorous Leafrollers refer to it, the Promised Land.

The USDA data sheet for fluoride lists raisins at 2.34 ppm, but

---

[67] For the record, my husband objects to this stereotype. I was about to delete it but then my editor gave it an "Amen." Now what?

as we've seen with other foods, those numbers have so many variables that putting stock in a government average is like taking the Queen of Heart's facial impressions at face value. Researchers at the University of Kansas measured five brands of California raisins and found fluoride levels as high as 5.2 ppm.[68] However, there is reason to believe that if you play raisin roulette long enough, you will stumble onto some raisins with much more fluoride than that.

The amount of fluoride in raisins depends on a number of factors including the quantity of pesticide used, the rate of dilution, timing of the application, humidity levels, rainfall, war rations, a government-sanctioned raisin mafia that could only exist in Wonderland, and current trends in baked goods.

As you can probably tell, there's a story here. It is reaching from beyond the grave to be told.[69] When I began digging into the topic of raisins and fluoride for this book, I unearthed a dark side of America's favorite dried fruit. Instead of telling the twisted tale to you here, I decided to post it online so it could have a wider audience. But here is the moral of the story. The sad history of fluoride and raisins demonstrates why your mother tried to teach you to always do your best to ensure your words are true. You repeat one little fib about fluoride being "safe and effective" and before you know it, you're not just a dentist or a bureaucrat anymore. You're a puppy killer.[70]

Humpty Dumpty sat on a wall,
Bones of fluoride—skin, joints and all.
Awful fish carcass, Tweedledodo said,
Let's poison cereal with raisins instead.

---

[68] Burgstahler, A. W., Robinson, M.A., "Fluoride in California wines and raisins," *Fluoride,* vol. 30, issue 3, 1997, pp. 142-146.

[69] Little Known Fact: The day I wrote this line, it was Halloween. Spooky, right?

[70] You can read the full story of raisins and fluoride at ProjectFree.Me/Raisins.

*****

Caterpillars Blowing Smoke

The food and beverages described in this chapter so far are the common sources of fluoride I came across during my experience of fluoroderma, but I would not be surprised if your list is different. You and I live on different pieces of earth. We eat diverse foods and breath distant air. It is entirely possible you will run into sources of fluoride I have not yet encountered. In those situations, you will need to do your own investigative work. But you already have access to all the resources any superhero needs to be successful: a nerdy sidekick like Internet and a superpower (i.e., your little layman brain).[71]

For example, raisins are all the rage right now, but perhaps you, being the enlightened raisin rebel that you now are, develop an affinity for dried apricots instead. *Viva la resistance!* If you ask Internet if cryolite can be used on apricots, she will take you to the EPA database for pesticide tolerances which confirms, as with grapes, fresh apricots have a residue tolerance for fluoride of 7 ppm. Does that mean dried apricots are high in fluoride? I don't know. Maybe? Sometimes? Not really? You will have to look at where your apricot stash is produced and then research pesticide usage reports for that region. Or contact the manufacturer. Or do some experiments on your skin to see how it reacts. Or just eat organic apricots instead.

The use of cryolite is not restricted to California and it's not reserved for dried fruit.[72] Cryolite is allowed to be applied to a variety of crops throughout the United States, including lettuce, berries, brussels sprouts, eggplant, kale, peaches, peppers, plums, tomatoes

---

[71] Since layman is a relative term, ALL of us have brains that are mostly layman (with maybe a little non-layman mixed in).

[72] For a map of cryolite use in the United States, see the cryolite page of the National Water Quality Program's Pesticide National Synthesis Project created by the U.S. Geological Survey (available at http://water.usgs.gov/nawqa/pnsp/usage/maps/compound_listing.php).

and more. My fluoroderma convinced me to switch to organic produce and therefore I do not have extensive experience on whether or not any of these foods cause breakouts. I still eat what I assume to be conventional produce at most restaurants. As long as they aren't steamed in fluoridated water, my skin doesn't seem to mind. (I should note, I am much more selective in choosing where I eat now that I know how food affects my acne. Most of my meals are prepared at home, but when eating out I try to limit my choices to restaurants with actual chefs who are cognizant of the quality of their raw ingredients.)

Fields, orchards, and vineyards aren't the only places fluoridated chemical warfare is waged in the name of mass produce. In the last decade, another avenue for fluoride-based pesticides has risen to the forefront of the American food supply. The story begins with the return of our favorite story-time character: raisins.

If you've ever seen the inside of a raisin warehouse, you know exactly what I am talking about. Whole species of invaders have risen up in San Joaquin Valley to seize humanity's hard-fought heaps of raisin booty. Dusky raisin moths, hairy fungus beetles, bark lice—these are just a few of the callous warriors caught looting our rightful raisin caches.[73] They covertly infiltrate our bunkers while the Raisin Reserves are sleeping, setting up shanty towns that attract predators of their own. Dedicated armies of brown ants dig impressive underground tunnel systems extending to depths of 3 feet or more to facilitate their mission of carrying off dead and dying larvae of storage moths stung by parasites. In springtime, surviving larvae pupate and emerge from the raisin depths.[74]

---

[73] For a fascinating read, see "Insects on Dried Fruit, Agriculture Handbook 464," Agricultural Research Service U.S. Department of Agriculture, 1975.

[74] "During one harvest, a beetle of the family Curculionidae, Dinocleus capillosus Csiki, was abundant in vineyards and later in the boxed raisins. The insects were about the same size and weight as Thompson Seedless raisins. Raisin-cleaning machinery did not remove them; expensive hand-sorting was necessary, accounting for the origin of the common phrase "one beetle for you, one beetle for you." SOURCE: "Insects on Dried Fruit, Agriculture Handbook 464," Agricultural Research Service U.S. Department of Agriculture, 1975, p. 9.

To combat enemy forces, in 2002, raisin handlers started using a toxic gas called ProFume to fumigate raisin bunkers. You are probably unfamiliar with ProFume unless you work in the industry, but you know its older sibling, Vikane. Since the early 1960s, Vikane has been the cornerstone of residential termite fumigation and is also occasionally used to control bedbugs and other infestations. Both Vikane and ProFume were developed by Dow AgroSciences using sulfuryl fluoride as the active ingredient.

As with cryolite, EPA considers fluoride as the toxicological endpoint of concern with sulfuryl fluoride, but unlike cryolite, there is no confusion over the fact that sulfuryl fluoride is highly toxic to humans. Even dentists can't find a way to dismiss the health effects experienced by people like the 37-year old woman found crawling out from under a termite fumigation tent in 2008, disoriented, vomiting, and three hours from death.[75] In 2015, Peyton McCaughey, a 10-year old boy in South Florida, suffered extensive brain damage after returning to his house which was recently fumigated with sulfuryl fluoride to kill termites.[76]

Despite its known toxicity, the EPA approved the use of sulfuryl fluoride on food products in 2002 with an Experimental Use Permit that allowed 12 ppm for fluoride on walnuts and 30 ppm on raisins.[77] (Dow had petitioned for an exemption to the requirement for a fluoride tolerance on raisins but EPA's Mathematics Department calculated 30 ppm as a fair compromise between 12 and infinity.) The United States needed an alternative to methyl bromide, another pesticide Dow produced, which was globally banned by the Vienna Convention's Montreal Protocol. If you refer back to our handy

---

[75] Schneir A, Clark RF, Kene M, Betten D. "Systemic fluoride poisoning and death from inhalational exposure to sulfuryl fluoride," *Clinical Toxicology*, vol. 46, issue 9, 2008, pp. 850-854.

[76] Ganim, Sara, "10-year-old hospitalized after termite fumigation," *CNN*, Sep 5, 2015.

[77] "Sulfuryl Fluoride; Temporary Pesticide Tolerances," Federal Register, Vol. 67, No. 26, February 7, 2002, pp. 5735-5740.

periodic chart from chapter three, you'll notice that bromine sits below fluorine in the halogen group. After learning their lesson with methyl bromide, most countries at least made an attempt to pursue less toxic pesticides in its place. But not in the United States. We decided to spray our snacks with termite fumigant instead.

In 2004, just two years after the Experimental Use Permit was approved for raisins and walnuts, sulfuryl fluoride was approved for widespread use as a food fumigant. Consequently, EPA set the highest levels of fluoride residue ever allowed on food in the United States, including 70 ppm for beans, 125 ppm for wheat flour, and *nine hundred* ppm for powdered eggs. At that point, why not just make scrambled eggs out of sodium fluoride powder? (This does not end well.[78]) Or eat a toothpaste sandwich?[79]

Consumer protection groups like the Fluoride Action Network, the Environmental Working Group, and Beyond Pesticides joined forces with a pro bono lawyer from American University to try to reverse EPA's approval of sulfuryl fluoride as a food fumigant. In 2011, after 8 years of effort, EPA was forced to admit that children were over-exposed to aggregate sources of fluoride. By their own calculations, they estimated that sulfuryl fluoride accounted for 3 percent of total fluoride exposure and thus they agreed to phase it out over a period of 3 years.

Realizing EPA was trapped by ineffable algorithms from its own Mathematics Department, Dow switched its focus to Congressional lobbies and managed to slip a sentence into President Obama's 1,000-page Farm Bill ordering EPA without explanation to ignore all non-pesticide sources of fluoride when calculating fluoride

---

[78] Little Known Fact: In 1942, a cook at Oregon State Hospital for the Insane made scrambled eggs for 467 mental patients using sodium fluoride (used for rat poison at the asylum) instead of powdered milk. It was an honest mistake, but 47 of the patients died by the next day. SOURCE: John, Finn J. D., "Horrifying asylum kitchen mix-up left dozens dead," *offbeat OREGON*, Nov 19, 2012.

[79] See ProjectFree.Me/Al-Bundy-Toothpaste-Sandwich/ (do not try this at home).

pesticide tolerances.[80] The sentence was added just a few days before the final vote, leaving little time for the public to organize opposition or for government politicians to understand what they were signing. Of course that did not keep them from signing it.

When Obama proudly signed the Farm Bill into law in February 2014, the United States became one of only two countries that allows sulfuryl fluoride to be sprayed on food.[81] With their market share safely in tact, the Dow Chemical Company then offloaded Dow AgroSciences, the division that produces Vikane and ProFume, in a sale to Douglas Products one year later. A Dow spokesperson claimed the reason for the sale was because the company "believes that this business segment has a greater opportunity to reach its full potential under a different owner. [And also, did you see what we just went through to get that sh** approved? Buy low, sell high, hold through tough times. Duh.]"[82]

With government actors writing the rules (as industry lobbyists whisper them their lines), it's easy to feel demoralized, disillusioned, and defeated. But let's not focus on them. Let's focus on *you*. You don't need to be a victim of the government's delusional approach to raisin-inspired chemical warfare. If the idea of eating termite fumigant does

---

[80] "Notwithstanding any other provision of law, the Administrator of the Environmental Protection Agency shall exclude nonpesticideal sources of fluoride from any aggregate exposure assessment required under section 408 of the Federal Food, Drug, and Cosmetic Act (21 U.S.C. 346a) when assessing tolerances associated with residues from the pesticide." SOURCE: "Regulation of Sulfuryl Fluoride," H.R. 2642, Public Law No. 113-79, Section 10015, Feb 7, 2014.

[81] For more information on how other countries handle sulfuryl fluoride for food-related fumigation, see "The Universal Consensus on Sulfuryl Fluoride = Keep It Away from Food," Fluoride Action Network, 2013.

[82] If you haven't figured this out yet, I am a pathological misquoter. It's a medical condition that results in a chemical compulsion to insert sass when called for, even if it means breaking the accepted rules of grammar. I wouldn't call it misquoting, though, it's more like quoting between the lines. If you have enjoyed said sass, please consider donating a few dollars to the legal defense fund I will surely need to defend myself from the pesticide journalists and spokespersons who published the boring original quote (sorry, Brad). If you missed the May 8th edition of *Pest Control Technology,* then you can read the original quote here: Harbison, Brad, "Dow to Sell Sulfuryl Fluoride to Douglas Products," *Pest Control Technology*, May 8, 2015.

not appeal to you, you have the option of buying organic. That probably means you will need to spend more money and might even have to change your shopping venues, but once you understand the health risk associated with raisin roulette—and produce poker in general—it is easier to find room in your budget.

When I first realized the negative effect fluoride was causing on my skin, I did not have a job and I was in debt from an upside-down mortgage for a house I could not live in. Organic food seemed needlessly expensive compared to what I was accustomed to buying, but my cystic acne was strong motivation to change my shopping habits. I watched basic cable on a 13" hand-me-down television and used a flip phone long after iPhones hit the market, but I managed to buy organic food because it was my priority.

If you suffer from cystic acne like I did, and have money to buy books to indulge your guilty obsession with raisin dramas, then I suspect organic food will be a priority for you too—especially now that you're privy to the long-concealed secret that diet causes acne (and sometimes other bad side effects, like death).

There are a few other sources of fluoride exposure you might run into besides diet. Pesticide manufacturers have discovered that fluoride is good at killing unwanted house guests, but it has many other utilities. As I mentioned in chapter one, fluoride can alter the melting point of metals but it can also make chemicals more durable, modify their propensity to dissolve in fats and oils, or increase the bioavailability of pharmaceuticals by enabling more of the dose to reach systemic circulation.

Approximately 20 percent of pharmaceuticals are estimated to contain fluoride,[83] including many of the top drugs such as Prozac, Paxil, Cipro, Flonase, and Lipitor to name just a few.[84] According to Manfred Schlosser, a professor of chemistry at the Swiss Federal

---

[83] Thayer, Ann M., "Fabulous Fluorine," *Chemical and Engineering News,* vol. 84, no. 23, Jun 5, 2006, pp. 15-24..

[84] For a more comprehensive list, see www.slweb.org/ftrcfluorinatedpharm.html.

Institute of Technology, a rule of thumb in medicinal chemistry is that "smuggling fluorine into a lead structure enhances the probability of landing a hit almost 10-fold."[85]

Drug manufacturers will tell you this type of fluoride is so stable it does not break down in the human body, and yet some studies clearly show elevated levels of fluoride in urine or blood following the use of fluoridated medication.[86]

Speaking of unintended bodily consequences, remember the Scotchgard debacle, when we realized the chemical 3M was marketing to save seat cushions from wine stains wasn't just accumulating in human tissue but could also be found in arctic polar bears who didn't care about their seat cushions and rarely even drink wine?[87] Fluoride was the culprit at that crime scene. Over a decade after banning the Scotchgard formula, we are still trying to figure out what exactly is going on with those fluoridated chemicals after they enter living bodies and how to clean them up.[88]

Perhaps you are familiar with the controversy surrounding

---

[85] Thayer, "Fabulous Fluorine."

[86] For examples, see the following:

Rioli, C. et al., "Relationship between serum concentrations of flecainide and fluoride in humans," *Bolletine Chimico Farmaceutico,* vol. 130, issue 7, Jul-Aug 1991, pp. 279-282.

Pradhan, K.M., et al. "Safety of ciprofloxacin therapy in children: magnetic resonance images, body fluid levels of fluoride and linear growth." Acta Paediatrica, vol. 84, issue 5, 1995, pp. 555-560.

Other examples available at fluoridealert.org/issues/sources/pharmaceuticals/.

[87] I say "rarely" because of this guy: www.thedrinksbusiness.com/2015/11/polar-bear-raids-bbc-film-crew-wine-supply/.

[88] For the backstory on 3M and Scotchgard, see "3M and Scotchgard: 'Heroes of Chemistry' or a 20-year coverup?" in Chemical Industry Archives, a project of the Environmental Working Group (available at www.chemicalindustryarchives.org/dirtysecrets/scotchgard/1.asp).

To give just one example of the Scotchgard legacy, see "Banned Scotchgard chemical still contaminating San Francisco seals" by Jane Kay, *Environmental Health News,* Jan 30, 2014.

non-stick cookware? Yes, the f-word is to blame there, too. The same super-strong fluoride bonds that keep wine from adhering to seat cushions also prevent other national emergencies such as eggs sticking to pans.[89] As their own internal documents attest, DuPont, the makers of Teflon, noticed as early as 1955 that "harmful compounds" were given off in the air when their nonstick pans were heated above 400 degrees Fahrenheit. They didn't bother telling anyone about it at the time because they weren't able to "duplicate in animal tests *the symptoms observed in humans*" (emphasis added because *really?!*).[90]

Besides releasing harmful contents into the air, non-stick coating can also add fluoride to the cooking contents. A study published in the *Journal of Dental Research* measured the fluoride content of water that had been boiled for 15 minutes in pots made of aluminum, stainless steel, pyrex, and Teflon.[91] The water boiled in Teflon contained three times more fluoride than any of the other samples.

Remember that time in the '80s when someone tried to explain to Romy and Michele that their supersized can of beloved hairspray was causing a hole in the ozone? It didn't make the film, but fluoride was in that scene and it was *awe-some*. DuPont first recognized the commercial potential of fluoride bonds when they created refrigerants by combining fluoride, chlorine, and carbon, known as chloro*fluoro*-carbons (CFCs). CFCs were used in aerosol cans, fire extinguishers, cleaning solvents and other products before they were banned by the Montreal Protocol, but they were largely replaced by hydro*fluoro*-

---

[89] You could go the old-fashioned route and use butter, but that's a topic for my next book.

[90] "Two types of reaction have been noted in humans as the result of accidental inhalation of the products of heated polymer. 1) a condition similar to metal fever; and 2) a condition in which there may be an irritation of the lungs leading to pulmonary edema." DuPont bulletin No. X-59a. As cited by Christopher Bryson in *The Fluoride Deception*, New York: Seven Stories Press, 2011, kindle location 4763-4764.

[91] Full, C.A., Parkins, F.M., "Effect of cooking vessel composition on fluoride." *Journal of Dental Research*, vol. 54, 1975, p. 192.

carbons and had already spawned an entire catalogue of other fluoride-based chemicals.

In addition to non-stick cookware and stain protectors, fluoride is still used in an assortment of products such as flame retardants, cosmetics, waterproof clothing, greasy food packaging, pizza boxes, and microwave popcorn bags. In May 2015, hundreds of scientists from around the world signed a document called the Madrid Statement published in *Environmental Health Perspectives* to warn of the severe health risks associated with the promiscuous use of fluorinated chemicals and to call for their restricted use and further study.[92]

In a response published in the same journal issue and written by a lawyer from the FluoroCouncil, a global organization representing the world's leading fluorotechnology companies, the industry admits the old fluoride chemicals they sold us for the last 50+ years were really bad and should definitely be removed from production, but they assure us the new and improved fluoride chemicals they are planning to sell us for the next 50+ years are "less toxic" and remain in living tissue and the atmosphere for "substantially shorter" periods of time.[93]

It's a tough call, but I say we go with the global community of independent scientists on this one.

---

[92] Blum, Arlene et al., "The Madrid Statement on Poly- and Perfluoroalkyl Substances (PFASs)," *Environmental Health Perspectives*, vol. 123, issue 5, May 2015.

Also see the corresponding Consumers' Guide to Highly Fluorinated Chemicals, available at GreenSciencePolicy.org/highly-fluorinated-chemicals/.

[93] Bowman, Jessica S., "Fluorotechnology Is Critical to Modern Life: The FluoroCouncil Counterpoint to the Madrid Statement," *Environmental Health Perspective*, vol. 123, issue 5, May 2015.

Jessica is a lawyer that represents the FluoroCouncil in Washington, D.C. To read the scientists' response to her statement, see Cousins, Ian et al., "Comment on 'Fluorotechnology Is Critical to Modern Life: The FluoroCouncil Counterpoint to the Madrid Statement,'" *Environmental Health Perspectives*, vol. 123, issue 7, 2015.

To read Jessica's response to their response, see Bowman, Jessica, "Response to "Comment on 'Fluorotechnology Is Critical to Modern Life: The FluoroCouncil Counterpoint to the Madrid Statement,'"" Environmental Health Perspectives, vol. 123, issue 7, 2015.

Realizing our modern lives are set in a piping hot bowl of toxic suey causes some people (*dad!*) to throw up their hands in defeat. "Something's gotta kill you eventually," they reason, "so you might as well eat poisoned popcorn." That's stupid. Don't do that. Unpoisoned popcorn is tastier anyway.[94] Other people roll their eyes at the word "toxin" and say dumb things like "if toxins scare you, stop eating."[95] Very helpful, thanks.

We live in an era when we know enough about chemistry to be dangerous but not enough to be wise. Most of us think someone out there is testing and regulating the safety of the manufactured chemicals staring back at us from the store shelves. We read product labels on carefully designed boxes and assume they tell the whole story, or at least the important parts. The reality is that the legislation regulating industrial chemicals in the United States, known as the Toxic Substances Control Act or TSCA (pronounced "tosca"), was passed into law in *nineteen seventy-six and hasn't been substantially updated since then.*

Much has happened since 1976. For starters, over half the current U.S. population was born, including me. The EPA banned asbestos because it causes cancer in humans and then unbanned asbestos because it causes lawsuits from industry attorneys. Polar bears settled with 3M for an undisclosed sum of sticky notes in exchange for their continued silence on the Scotchgard incident. CFCs, PCBs, PFOAs, PFOSs, P. Diddy and then just Diddy except in the U.K.,[96] all these experiences offer us lessons we could have been using

---

[94] Here's how to make the best popcorn you will ever eat. Heat a generous spoonful of coconut oil in a large pot or a stovetop popcorn maker. Add 3 kernels of organic popcorn and cover the pot. When the kernels pop, add a 1/2 cup of kernels to the heated oil. Shake the pan or rotate the popcorn turner as the rest of the kernels pop. Sprinkle with sea salt and drench in melted butter from pastured cows. Snuggle on couch and watch *Food, Inc.* or *Elf*, as appropriate for the season.

[95] For example, www.science20.com/science_20/thanksgiving_chemophobia_if_ toxins_scare_you_stop_eating-118737.

[96] https://en.wikipedia.org/wiki/Diddy_(DJ)

to improve our approach to industrial chemical regulation. Instead, we keep doing it the same old way we've been doing it since 1976.[97] That's government status quo in inaction. Again.

Our current paralysis in chemical regulation goes back even further than the 1970s. When government bureaucrats implemented the Toxic Substances Control Act, they decided to grandfather in 62,000 preexisting industrial chemicals solely in the name of status quo —most of them were never even tested for adverse health effects. As a result, when you use a common household product to *"freshen"* air, *"soften"* fabric, *"dissolve"* stains, etc., you are likely relying on the scientific sophistication of a 1950s businessman to guarantee your safety and the marketing prowess of the 1950s adman he hired to inculcate the need for the product deep into your psyche.

If you are accustomed to picking any product off the shelf and giving it a try, then this information *should* have a dramatic effect on your purchasing habits. But I know it can be hard to rewire your thought process when all these products seem perfectly normal. It's like when I tried to convince my parents they shouldn't trust email from random strangers (or phone calls, *mom!*) and then visit the websites they suggest. Things might seem fine at the time, but chances are some nasty code made its way into your system—or worse—and your error in judgment will eventually catch up with you. The same is true with our naive trust in industrial chemicals, except when the time comes you won't be able to dump your body's old operating system and switch to a Mac.[98]

To be fair to my parents, everyone succumbs to naivety in one form or another. Our brains simply weren't designed to rethink every

---

[97] A TSCA Modernization Act was introduced to Congress in 2015 but industry lobbyists have been hard at work ensuring their interests are protected. Even if it does pass, the likelihood is slim that it will enact the change needed. The details of the proposed legislation (along with those of the existing TSCA rules) are so frustrating and boring I don't even feel like getting into it, but you can read more about them at www.ewg.org/key-issues/toxics/chemical-policy.

[98] Unless you believe in reincarnation. Ask Internet about "old souls Amazon." What?!

wheel we come across. That's the beauty of technology and human society in general, but it can also limit us to the widely-accepted beliefs of the time. To help smooth things over with my parents, I'll give an example from my own collection of dumb-things-I've-done.

One year, my unit at FBI Headquarters was moved to a different office and everyone was cleaning the Hoover-era crud from their new cubicles. A few times a day, I heard a loud *psssssst* coming from my coworkers' cubes. I eventually figured out they were using cans of "compressed air" to clean the keys between their keyboards. I had never heard of such an invention but I thought "Golly gee, Mr. Businessman, a can of crisp mountain air to dislodge the cookie crumbs inside the crevices of my keyboard? Gee whiz, thanks! What will you come up with next." As I pulled the trigger, my naivety quickly dissipated when the can turned ice cold in my hand. *Huh?* What kind of white witch cleaning devilry is this? Plain air doesn't do *that*.

Later that evening, Internet hooked me up with a keyboard cleaning data sheet written by two smartypants named Shirli and Larry who work for the City of Seattle. They patiently explained to me that "compressed air" isn't a bottled ocean breeze that propels itself onward full of nothing but sea scent and miracles. The brand of keyboard cleaner we were using was composed of a hydro*fluoro*carbon called HFC-152a. The fluoride-based chemical is also used as a refrigerant which explains why the can turned cold when I pressed the trigger. According to Shirli and Larry, HFC-152a is a flammable greenhouse gas and causes Central Nervous System depression leading to headaches and fatigue.

Eureka! Shirli and Larry had hit on something. As my coworkers were diligently tidying up their personal corners of Hoover Heaven, many of them started complaining of headaches, depressed immunity, and poor ventilation in our new workspace. An inspector was assigned to assess if the room was up to code. What are the chances he tested for hydrofluorocarbon? I gave Shirli and Larry's data sheet to my government point of contact, but he just put it with the other papers in the papers-to-be-routed-to-the-routing-box box. I am still waiting to hear back about it. Not long afterwards, my team was moved to a new Unit in our original workspace (which was not unusual given the government's well-known fondness for a rousing round of musical chairs—*so fun!* Even Shirli likes it).

Like my coworkers, I too experienced headaches while working in the new office before my childlike preconceptions of canned air were crushed, convincing me to find a way to be absent from my workspace until I was officially moved to a new desk. I don't recall hydrofluorocarbon affecting my acne, but I don't know what my skin would look like if I continued to inadvertently sniff chemical keyboard cleaner on a daily basis or if I lived next to an "air" factory.

I am bringing up the topic of fluoridated chemicals not because I have the answers but because you and I need to be asking the questions, instead of relying on 1950s businessmen and EPA's Question Department. Under the current TSCA regulations, EPA has 90 days to decide if a new chemical poses an "unreasonable risk" to public health, otherwise the product moves on to the marketing teams for an expert makeover before batting its eyelashes at you from retail shelves. The requisite catch-22 built into TSCA is that companies aren't required to test their new chemicals, and EPA regulators don't have the resources to do it themselves. Unless a company volunteers to test their chemicals and then provides derogatory information about them to EPA, the new chemical won't trigger the EPA's initial threshold for testing. So as long as there's no testing, there's no reason for further testing.

The method we've been relying on to gauge the safety of industrial chemicals in the United States for the last 40 years has been "don't test, don't tell." As long as no one asks if the chemicals are safe, we won't need to tell anyone they're poison because *no one will know if they are or not.*

A TSCA Modernization Act is finally floating around Congress, but industry spent over $64 million lobbying Washington last year (2014).[99] Companies like DuPont, 3M, and Dow Chemicals are all a little too happy with the proposed bill not to raise suspicions.

It is unlikely the chemical scene in the U.S. will change fast enough for you and me to benefit. If we don't want to be collateral damage, we will need to be discerning consumers instead. Good thing we've been exercising our little layman brains for just such a challenge. The government's policy is that industrial chemicals are innocent until proven guilty, but that doesn't mean it has to be our policy too. Unless a chemical product has a solid track record of—I don't know, let's say a few hundred years—then I think it's only prudent based on historical experience to be a little skeptical of it.

An obvious place to start is with chemicals that enter your body through your mouth, nose, skin, eyes, ears, scalp, lady parts, man parts, and whatnot.[100] Your Internet sidekick is happy to provide more information on any products you care to ask her about. The Environmental Working Group's shopping guides are excellent resources for safety information on cosmetics, cleaning products, sunscreen, bug spray, and other chemical concoctions that have made themselves necessities in our modern lives. Internet will even arrange for healthier options to be shipped directly to your doorstep by connecting you with online retailers who specialize in household products that are safer than the ones at Walmart and less expensive than Whole Foods. For some informational resources to get you started, visit **ProjectFree.Me/Skincare**.

In many cases, you probably don't even need a chemical product to fulfill the task at hand. To demonstrate, Shirli and Larry put their heads together and came up with an excellent list of safe alternatives to chemical keyboard cleaners, including inexpensive

---

[99] For background information on the current political effort to overhaul TSCA, see www.opensecrets.org/news/issues/chemical/.

[100] The parts on a whatnot are hard to generalize. Jim Henson explains it well. Ask YouTube.

keyboard vacuums that plug into your USB port, keyboard brushes and microfiber dusters, manual air blowers that look like turkey basters (Larry insisted on including a picture), and the ingenious method of turning your keyboard upside down to shake out debris. Scotchgard, Teflon, Static Guard, Febreze, Magic Wrinkle Releaser (it's not bottled magic, I checked)... Do we really need any of these products? Are they worth the risk? You know what Shirli and Larry would say, and they can be very persuasive.[101]

*****

A Jabberwock Among Us[102]

I hope you don't mind. This chapter ended up being a *teensy* bit longer than I anticipated. I blame those mimsy raisins.[103] But not to worry, we are finally getting around to the last major sources of fluoride you are likely to encounter in modern life as I know it. To bring the story full gyre, we'll end this chapter with a discussion of other sources of fluoride forced upon us directly by uffish dentists.

We already talked about the fluoride that gimbles its way into our diet from the water supply, but how are we affected by the continual use of fluoridated water that fills our showers, sinks, bath tubs, hot tubs, swimming pools, steam rooms, humidifiers, dialysis machines, colonic machines, enema bags, fish tanks, koi ponds, and borogove baths? The dentists haven't gotten around to studying these

---

[101] In the Kindle version of this book, there is a very persuasive graphic here. You can view it at ProjectFree.Me/not-bottled-magic.

[102] Jabberwock is derived from the anglo-saxon word for *wocor*, meaning "offspring" or "fruit," combined with *jabber*, meaning "excited and voluble discussion." Therefore a jabberwock signifies "the result of much excited and voluble discussion." I find it a fitting title for this sub-chapter.

[103] For a description of unfamiliar words in this section, see https://en.wikipedia.org/wiki/Jabberwocky.

avenues of fluoride exposure yet, and when they do I have a vorpal feeling they aren't going to do a snicker-snack job of it.

I'm happy to report that we can cross dialysis machines off our list of sources of fluoride exposure we need to worry about. Unfortunately, dialysis patients had to learn this lesson the hard way. I don't have any experience with dialysis machines, but from what Internet tells me, they were modified to filter out fluoride when doctors in the 1970s noticed dentists' infatuation with the F-drug had condemned frumious kidney patients to the accumulation of large amounts of fluoride in their bones and blood, leading to a mome bone disorder called osteomalacia.[104]

But what about the other means of fluoride exposure mentioned above? Even though we've been bathing our babies in fluoridated water for the last seventy years, I was not able to find any U.S. studies or statistics on the dermal absorption of the hydrofluorosilicic acid contained in the water supply. Reports of skin reactions from toothpaste and fluoridated steroid creams show that topical contact with fluoride can cause acne. The question is, at what concentration of fluoride are we affected? I will tell you my experience, but this is one of those questions that might require some tulgey investigative work on your part.

At the moment, my husband and I are temporarily living in an apartment outside Washington, D.C. where the water is fluoridated at 0.7 ppm. I am able to maintain clear skin even though I regularly shower and wash my hands in fluoridated water. However, when I first diagnosed my fluoroderma I lived in a condo fluoridated at 1.0 ppm and my acne did not heal completely until I moved to a non-fluoridated neighborhood. Perhaps if I had stayed in Fluorideville long enough I would have eventually been able to live there without my skin burbling, but at the time it seemed like the amount of fluoride they added to the water was too much for my chortled skin to handle,

---

[104] For more information and additional references, see www.fluoridealert.org/studies/kidney04/.

even though I was limiting my exposure as much as I knew how.

Based on these past experiences, my current approach is to minimize my exposure to topical sources of fluoride when possible without being obsessive or outgrabive about it. I don't worry about water touching my face in the shower, but I don't intentionally slithy it in, either.

In my experience, fluoride exposure from the shower is the trickiest source to avoid. It is possible to filter fluoride from your shower but it's not an easy fix because standard shower filters don't remove fluoride. For more information, see **ProjectFree.Me/Fluoride-Filters**. Since my primary residence in Florida is not fluoridated, my approach is simply to not spend as much time in the shower anytime I suspect the water from the faucet might be fluoridated.

A study of fluoride and sodium lauryl sulfate (SLS), a chemical found in a variety of cleansers and shampoos, found that SLS increased fluoride absorption in the mouth by nine percent.[105] Does it increase the absorption of fluoride through the skin, too? I don't know and I don't know if anyone else knows either. It appears those studies have not been conducted.

Other avenues of topical fluoride exposure are much easier to avoid. You can wear gloves while doing the dishes, and it's only a small inconvenience to wash your face with bottled water instead of water from the faucet. When I lived in Newport where they added particularly high amounts of fluoride, I remember washing my face with tap water and feeling a brillig, burning sensation on my skin. The experience convinced me to switch to using bottled water even though I knew nothing about fluoride at the time. I now wash my face with bottled water whenever I'm traveling.

Washing your face with bottled water isn't weird. The frabjous Cameron Diaz does it, too. Contrary to widespread reports in the

---

[105] Barkvoll, P. "Plasma F Levels Following Intake of NaF in Combination with Sodium Lauryl Sulphate," Abstracts of Posters, *Journal of Dental Research*, vol. 69, 1990, p. 827.

media, she uses an assortment of brands, not just Evian (that would be weird). In her recent book, *The Body Book*, Cameron describes how she suffered from chronic acne even as an adult, just like I did. Pictures show it was concentrated around her mouth and chin, just like mine.[106] Also like me, she tried all the popular treatments on the market—oral, topical, even the harshest prescriptions—but nothing worked for long.

At 30 years old, she had a health awakening and started being conscious of the quality of the food she was putting into her body. (Wait, am I Cameron Diaz?) She attributes her recovery from adult acne to the healthy home-cooked meals that replaced her fast-food addiction. Like Cordain's paleo dieters, Cameron explains her skin wasn't completely healed after she stopped eating tove burgers, barbecued rath ribs, and fried jubjub nuggets, but it was significantly better.[107] Whose wouldn't be? I don't doubt that her diet is greatly improved after ditching fast food, but I suspect the change in her acne was because she happened to eliminate significant sources of fluoride at the same time.[108]

While I tolerate showering and washing my hands in fluoridated water, baths are a different story. I haven't conducted any scientific studies on this, but to my little layman brain it seems as if there would be a difference between standing in a shower where the water is obliged by gravity to constantly move towards the drain like rain on a wabe, versus submerging your body in a pool of water for 20 to 40 minutes (or longer) while you're just taunting the water to move inwards.

---

[106] "Cameron Diaz Reveals Adult Acne Struggle: 'I Always Felt Really Bad About Myself,'" *Radar Online*, Dec 21, 2013.

[107] *Ibid.*

[108] If anyone can convince Cameron to read this book, I will give both you and Cameron a free t-shirt of your choosing featuring any of the following popular topics: Shirli and Larry's Guide to Musical Chairs, the logo for EPA's Mathematics Department (don't worry, it's sporty), or the latest ad for fried jubjub nuggets. Same applies for Emma Stone and Katy Perry who also struggle with adult acne and are equally frabjous.

In a study published in the *Journal of Public Health,* a research group led by Halina Brown, a toxicologist from the Massachusetts Department of Environmental Protection, analyzed the dermal absorption of various contaminants (not fluoride) and found that absorption through the skin accounted for 29 to 91 percent of the total dose. Whoa there, Halina. That is a serious observation. The team concluded that "skin absorption of contaminants in drinking water has been underestimated and that ingestion may not constitute the sole or even primary route of exposure."[109] Again, whoa.

If the CDC ever starts to wonder about the dermal absorption of the only chemical intentionally added to public water supplies because of its long-term effect on the human body, Brown's article provides some helpful tips for designing such a test. First, she points out that most researchers who conduct dermal studies of this nature tend to oversimplify matters (cough, *dentists*) by soaking their subjects' hands in a test solution and then measuring either the amount of the chemical excreted in their urine and breath, or the change in the chemical's concentration in the test solution. Furthermore, these studies typically involve manxome middle-aged man hands. Again, I haven't done any experiments to be sure of this, but it seems like they would absorb contaminants at a different rate than would beamish baby-aged ballerina hands, to give just one example.

Speaking of scrotums, Brown explains that hands aren't the proper limb to be using for these experiments since the epidermis on the hands is a greater barrier to penetration than other parts of the body. Scrotums, on the other hand, are more permeable than hands, are available on most test subjects used for modern medical studies, and are easily submerged due to their dangling topography. As Brown states, "Penetration through the scrotum, in fact, is estimated to be 100 per cent, as compared to 8.6 per cent for the forearm."

---

[109] Brown, H. S., Bishop, D. R., and Rowan, C. A. "The role of skin absorption as a route of exposure for volatile organic compounds (VOCs) in drinking water." *American Journal of Public Health,* vol. 74, issue 5, 1984, pp. 479–484.

Other factors Brown cites that affect the rate of dermal absorption include damage to the skin (such as sunburn, cuts, jock itch, etc.), a history of skin conditions that deplete the stratum corneum (such as eczema, psoriasis, crabs, etc.), previous exposure, nutrition, ratio of body fat, current hydration, chemical composition of the skin, temperature and pH of the solution, and also the lipophilicity, polarity, volatility, solubility, molecular weight, and carbon number of the chemical in question, as well as the presence of various other chemical compounds that act as accelerants or otherwise enhance permeability.

Even if all these factors are accounted for, Brown reminds researchers that some chemical compounds are "distributed slowly and may be sequestered in the body for relatively long periods," meaning that they might be absorbed by the body and still not show up in breath or urine 24 hours later (cough, *fluoride*).

Once dentists have created a dermal study for fluoridated water keeping all these factors in mind, to really do their due diligence they'll then need to conduct studies to account for greater rates of other routes of absorption, including aural (through the ears), nasal (up the nose), sublingual (under the tongue), buccal (inside of the cheeks), and orbital (I don't know this one—is it the butt?).[110] Until all those studies are done for various age groups and ethnicities in both males and females, it's hard to estimate exactly how much fluoride seeps into our bodies at bath time. But seep it does.

In the early 1930s, while American dentists were daydreaming of ways to save the world by turning tap water into mouthwash, European researchers were experimenting with fluoride for other motivations. They noticed that fluoride inhibits thyroid function (an effect we covered earlier, in Chapter 42), so they started studying the use of fluoride to treat patients with overactive thyroids.

---

[110] This is a rhetorical question. I don't really need to know the answer. Please don't email me about this unless you go by the name of Halina Brown (middle name: Szejnwald). Thank you for your cooperation on this matter.

Researchers in Austria, Germany, Italy, and France published research describing their experiments treating hyperthyroidism through fluoride therapy. I have not been able to find full texts of these studies and even the abstracts I've located aren't in English, but from what I can gather through Google Translate and other bits of information from Internet, some of the European researchers successfully lowered thyroid activity through the use of fluoridated *baths*.[111] In an interview on Joe Mercola's website, one source claims the baths only needed to last for 20 minutes to have an effect with water fluoridated at 4 to 5 ppm.[112] This concentration is significantly higher than current levels in the U.S., but some of us bathe for longer than 20 minutes, plus we've been bathing in, drinking, and eating fluoride since our baby ballerina years (or baby ballerino years, for the gents).[113]

Based on the limited information available about dermal absorption of fluoridated water, here is my approach to full-body submergence situations. Being a health nut, I naturally love detox baths of all sorts, but I *never* take baths in fluoridated water. I'm sure you would probably survive a fluoridated bath now and then if you are lucky,[114] but for me it's not worth the additional exposure. I would not be able to enjoy it anyway, knowing what I know about fluoride.

Also, I rarely swim in pools or soak in hot tubs other than my

---

[111] If you want to investigate this topic further, see ProjectFree.Me.References for links to some of the articles by European researchers who experimented with fluoride to treat hypothyroidism.

[112] Mercola, Joseph. "Non-Organic Foods Blast Your Body With Up to 180 Times the Fluoride in Drinking Water," Interview with Jeff Greene at Mercola.com, Feb 4, 2012.

[113] Spell check keeps telling me ballerino is not a word but it *is* a word. According to Wikipedia, "In Italian, a ballerina is a female who typically holds a principal title within a ballet company; the title for equally ranked males is ballerino." C'mon, spell check. This is an important gender issue. Think of how annoying auto-correct must be for all the ballerinos out there. This issue needs to be addressed.

[114] ;) <—to indicate I am being facetious here in case dentists try to take this quote out of context. Do you think dentists get the meaning of winky face? Never mind. Of course they do. They probably use it all the time, as in: fluoride is safe and effective. ;)

own. At our house in Florida, we are fortunate to have a saltwater pool and hot tub in our backyard, a setup that is not uncommon amongst Floridians. I do swim in the ocean, however, and "gotcha" dentists might point out that ocean water contains fluoride—they're really up on their natural fluoride sources. But as I mentioned previously, seawater contains a different composition of fluoride than the smokestack variety they choose to add to the public water supply (*gotcha!*). It also contains a lot of other minerals not found in tap water, any of which could affect how fluoride is absorbed by living tissue.

To be clear, I have absolutely no idea how much fluoride is contained in your typical pool water or if it is absorbed into the body. This is just how I, as a person living with fluoroderma, choose to handle these situations based on the limited information at hand and my preexisting dislike of public pools and hot tubs.

If reading those last few paragraphs made your heart sink at the thought of losing precious "me time" in the home spa, I'm sorry. This is clearly your dentist's fault. But since I hate seeing you this way, I will let you in on a secret. There is a frabjous alternative I am planning to suggest to you in the very next chapter. I will keep it a surprise for now, but if you're like me it will leave you shouting *Callooh! Callay!* from the highest branch of the nearest TumTum tree.

Before we get there, however, there are a few last tricks you should be aware of that the Cult of Dental Fluoride has been known to use to sneak their venerated element into your everyday life. Like any large-scale religion, various sects have arisen tailored to the temperaments and habits of local practitioners.

While the orthodox fluoride tradition developed in the United States elevates the role of dental clergy over the flock, emphasizing the water-into-mouthwash miracle, sects in other parts of the world have a more salt-of-the-earth interpretation of fluoride scripture. In one sect, individual practitioners are welcomed into a priesthood of all believers as they perform a little fluoride miracle with every sprinkle of the family salt shaker. The sect originated in Switzerland in 1955 when a

Swiss gynecologist pioneered the addition of fluoride to table salt. It took several decades to catch on, as these things often do, but because of a historical monopoly on the salt trade in Swiss cantons (a local government structure—you knew bureaucrats had to be involved somehow), most of the salt produced in Switzerland is now fluoridated.[115]

The practice of adding fluoride to salt was replicated to a limited extent in neighboring countries in Europe. Usually it is limited to home salt shakers, enabling individuals to have the option to faithfully sprinkle pesticide directly on their food or not, as desired.

According to an article published in *Schweiz Monatsschr Zahnmed,*[116] as of 2006 the following European countries allow fluoride to be added to salt (the number in parentheses is the percent of household salt that is fluoridated): Austria (6%), Czech Republic (15%), France (65%), Germany (67%), Slovakia (unknown), Spain (10%), and Switzerland (88%).[117] Belgium bans fluoridated salt because it is poison, while in the Netherlands it is only produced for export.[118] Fluoride missionaries spread the sect to countries in Latin America and the Caribbean, especially Jamaica, Costa Rica, Colombia, Mexico, Peru, and Uruguay.[119] The sect is rare in Africa and Asia although the World Health Organization sponsored a few programs in areas of Madagascar, Laos, and Vietnam.[120]

---

[115] Marthaler, Thomas M., "Overview of salt fluoridation in Switzerland since 1955, a short history," *Schweiz Monatsschr Zahnmed*, vol. 115, 2005, pp. 651–655.

[116] Translation: My Little Swiss Monster Named Zahnmed. As you can tell from the footnotes in this section, *Schweiz Monatsschr Zahnmed* is a religious magazine used to discuss historical and theological aspects of salt fluoridation. Zahnmed must be the name of their fluoride deity or something.

[117] Gotzfried F. "Legal aspects of fluoride in salt, particularly within the EU." *Schweiz Monatsschr Zahnmed*, vol. 116, 2006, pp. 371-375.

[118] *Ibid.*

[119] Gillespie, George M., Baez, Ramon. "Development of salt fluoridation in the Americas," *Schweiz Monatsschr Zahnmed*, vol. 115, 2005, pp. 663-669.

[120] Petersen, P.E.., Phantumvanit, P. "Toward Effective Use of Fluoride in Asia," *SAGE Publications*, vol. 24, issue 2, 2012.

A disparate sect of believers shun fluoridated water and salt altogether and instead cling to prophecy about a land overflowing with milk and fluoride. In parts of Bulgaria, Chile, China, Peru, Russia, Thailand, and the United Kingdom, fluoride is added to milk (usually powdered frankenmilk) for distribution to school systems and food assistance programs aimed at defenseless children.[121]

Lest we become caught up in the religious fervor and forget our fluoride facts, just because these programs exist in small enclaves around the world does not mean they are safe or effective. According to a Cochrane review of milk fluoridation programs, there is no quality evidence that fluoridated milk prevents dental caries and no information on the potential health hazards.[122] A Cochrane review of fluoridated salt was proposed in 2009, in part by two WHO dentists, but from what I can gather it was never published.[123] (My investigator instincts tell me there's a story there, but I will leave it for someone else to tell.)

There is one last situation in which you will need to be on high guard against fluoride exposure. It's the most dangerous source referenced in this entire chapter, but you will likely encounter it only once or twice per year and in just one place: your dentist's chair.

Fluoride gel and other fluoridated dental treatments such as varnishes, rinses, polishes, etc. contribute not just to chronic fluoride toxicity but are also a primary source of *acute* fluoride toxicity. Fluoride gels were introduced in the 1960s without any clinical evidence of being safe or effective.[124] Who needs evidence when you have faith?

---

[121] "Milk Fluoridation," Alliance for a Cavity Free Future at AllianceforaCavityFreeFuture.org.

[122] Yeung, C.; Chong, L.; Glenny, A., "Fluoridated milk for preventing tooth decay," Cochrane Database of Systematic Reviews, Sep 2015.

[123] Gillespie, G.; Baez, R., et al. "Salt fluoridation for preventing dental caries," Cochrane Database of Systematic Reviews, Jan 2009.

[124] Ekstrand J. "Pharmacokinetic aspects of topical fluorides," *Journal of Dental Research*, vol. 66, issue 5, 1987, pp. 1061-1065 as cited at fluoridealert.org/issues/dental-products/gels/).

It took dentists a couple decades to notice that a dangerous portion of the 12,300 ppm of fluoride contained in dental gel was finding its way into their patients' bloodstreams, causing spikes 100 times greater than normal levels and sometimes lasting up to 14 hours following treatment.[125]

Even when it's not swallowed, fluoride's high acidity enhances its entry directly into the bloodstream from buccal and sublingual absorption (and possibly orbital??), bypassing what drug researchers refer to as "first pass metabolism" in the digestive system.[126] This is why many people experience stomach pain, nausea, headaches, and vomiting shortly after their dentist gives them a free toothbrush and then gallumphs off to poison another unsuspecting patient like a whiffling bandersnatch in flight.

What's that you say? Your cousin's best friend's sister is a dental hygienist, and she says none of her patients ever threw up after a dental cleaning? Well, that evidence sounds anecdotal so let's ask Internet about it to see what other anekdota we can find. Internet: kids vomiting fluoride. Go...

That was easy. Here are just a few accounts from the first forum I clicked on.

*****

---

[125] Ekstrand, J., Koch, G. "Systemic fluoride absorption following fluoride gel application," *Journal of Dental Research*, vol. 59, issue 6, 1980, p. 1067.

[126] Whitford, G.M., et al. "Fluoride absorption through the hamster cheek pouch: a pH-dependent event." *Journal of Applied Toxicology*, vol. 2, issue 6, Dec 1982, pp. 303-306 (as cited at fluoridealert.org/studies/gels01/).

Metasequoia writes at "My Kids Were Poisoned Today - Who to Write To?" on Mothering.com:[127] Dd1 (8) & Dd2 (5) had their teeth cleaned while Ds (2) had his cleaned… As soon as we walked out of the building, Dd1 said, "Mommy, that stuff they put on my teeth made my belly feel yucky & gave me a headache." Then we got in the car & Dd2 started complaining that she felt yucky. Less than 5 minutes later, Ds was vomiting all over himself. The girls continued to complain & Dd2 threw up all over herself & her car seat. Dd1 made it home, but barely, vomiting in the front yard. I called their dentist's office & asked what it was that they used that would cause all three of my children to vomit & they said that "fluoride sometimes causes kids to feel sick to their stomachs." I am BEYOND FURIOUS!!! Why, in their minds, is this a reasonable reaction???!!

> **username not worth mentioning because she blames the kids replies:** How did they get sick to their stomach from topical flouride?! Surely your 8 year old wasn't swallowing was she? If she swallowed the flouride, it's not exactly the doctor's fault...he was doing his job

> [*Author's note:* Sorry, I just have to jump in here. Honey, did you not notice Dd2 is 5 and Ds is only 2? Are they also to blame for swallowing fluoride? Plus, things get into your body through other routes besides your stomach. You are posting on a mothering forum so I suspect you already figured this out, I'm just reminding you.]

> **latinmom replies:** It's very easy to have this kind of reaction. Some kids can't help but swallow a little. I refuse it for my kids and myself-I have exactly this reaction, and I don't swallow any that I know of.

---

[127] Comments posted at "My Kids Were Poisoned Today - Who to Write To?" by Metasequoia at Mothering.com, May 22, 2008 (available at www.mothering.com/forum/14-activism-news/902528-my-kids-were-poisoned-today-who-write.html).

CalaRei replies: Eugh. I always threw up because of fluoride treatments. I think once I even threw up ON him, through those gummy trays. I would just sit there and cry and cry until the time was up, and then frantically wash out my mouth repeatedly.

another blame the kid replies: I am a hygienist. I only had one kid throw up from a Fluoride treatment because he swallowed when I had told him not to. Other than that, I never had a kid throw up.

[*Author's note:* Notice how the fluoridation faithful sometimes capitalize fluoride? That's a gang sign. You also aren't supposed to speak fluoride's real name out loud. Us heathens don't even know what it is.][128]

zooeyzoo replies: Thank you to the OP who posted this. I was getting nasaus all the time lately and couldn't figure out why until I looked at my toothpaste. I changed to a flouride free toothpaste and it's gone. Looks like I'm sensitive to it too even though I only use it topically.

breeder replies: I still remember vomiting from flouride treatments when I was a kid. Poor kiddos. :(

*****

So you can tell your cousin's best friend's sister that it looks like vomiting from dental cleanings is a real thing. Death from dental cleanings is also a real thing. It doesn't happen often, but at least one incident was reported by the *New York Times* on May 24, 1974 when a

---

[128] Is it Fluoristan? Zahnmed? I'm dying to know. If you have ideas for what the secret cult name for fluoride might be among dental devotees, please share them on Twitter using #FCultExposed. There just might be a free religious t-shirt at stake here (you get to pick the sect).

Brooklyn boy named William Kennerly died after swallowing a fluoride varnish the hygienist painted on his teeth.[129] She was engrossed in conversation during the treatment and when she handed him a cup of water afterwards, she forgot to tell him he was supposed to use it to rinse and spit, not to drink. Being that it was his first visit to the dentist, 3-year old William did what any 3-year old child would do and drank the cup of water the healthcare professional handed him.

When William started sweating, vomiting, and complaining of headache and dizziness before leaving the doctor's office, his mother appealed to the dentist for help but was told not to worry because it was just a routine treatment. Unsatisfied with his answer, she immediately took her son to the ambulatory pediatric care unit nearby where they waited for over two hours to see a doctor. She thought William had fallen asleep in the waiting room, but he had actually slipped into a coma and died a few hours later after being transported to a local hospital. At the supreme court hearing that followed, a doctor testified that William's life might have been saved if the dentist had simply given him a glass of salt water to counteract the fluoride in his digestive system.

Apparently dentists still aren't aware of the dangers of fluoridated gel because they have never studied them. In 2015, the Cochran Oral Health Group reviewed the available research on the safety and effectiveness of fluoride gels for preventing tooth decay.[130] Of course they found that most of the evidence on fluoride's effectiveness was of low quality, moderate at best. But they also concluded, "There is little information on adverse effects or on acceptability of treatment. Future trials should include assessment of potential adverse effects."

Let me repeat their conclusion in more everyday terms. Even

---

[129] McFadden, Robert D. "$750,000 Given In Child's Death In Fluoride Case," *The New York Times,* Jan 20, 1979 (available at www.fluoridealert.org/articles/kennerly/).

[130] Marinho, V.C.C. et al. "Fluoride gels for preventing dental caries in children and adolescents." Cochrane Database of Systematic Reviews, Jun 2015.

though fluoride gels have been used in American dental clinics for over *fifty years* on people who are literally vomiting in the car on the way home, few studies have been carried out on their adverse health effects. Who needs studies when you have faith?

When you lie down in the dentist's chair, *you* are relying on faith, too. Every time you visit the dentist, it is important to remember that today's dentists are playing with an element more dangerous than fire. They are playing with fluoride.[131]

> *"It was all very well to say 'Drink me,' but the wise little Alice was not going to do that in a hurry. 'No, I'll look first,' she said, 'and see whether it's marked "poison" or not'... she had never forgotten that, if you drink much from a bottle marked 'poison,' it is almost certain to disagree with you, sooner or later. However, this bottle was not marked 'poison,' so Alice ventured to taste it, and finding it very nice, (it had, in fact, a sort of mixed flavour of cherry-tart, custard, pine-apple, roast turkey, toffee, and hot buttered toast,) she very soon finished it off."*
>
> —Lewis Carroll, *Alice's Adventures in Wonderland*

---

[131] Visit **ProjectFree.Me/Fluoride** to receive a 1-page Quick Guide on the sources of fluoride described in this chapter.

5

HEALING BREAKOUTS OVERNIGHT

"Even miracles take a little time."
—Cinderella's Fairy Godmother

SKINCARE PRODUCTS ONLY PLAY A BIT PART IN OUR STORY. If you develop your skill at avoiding the fluoride sources described in the previous chapter, you won't have to worry about breakouts anymore no matter what your skincare routine is. You will be one of those people who can sleep in makeup (or if you're like me, dog saliva) for three weeks straight without so much as a stressed pore. But there must be something that can be done to help the poor unfortunate souls who are in the midst of a fluoroderma flareup.

Until you learn how to dust off all the traces of dentist fingerprints in your daily life, this chapter offers a little touch of magic to get you through any existing or future breakouts quickly, sometimes as fast as overnight. But first, a spell has been cast and we need to break it. Potent potions will emerge from competing cauldrons. Bad witches will be outed and good witches will come to our aid. And when we finally reach the start of our story, we will all be transformed from merfolk into humans.

*****

A Poisoned Part of Your World

The spells cast by the beauty industry are so powerful and pervasive that it is hard to find a modern woman who does not take a bite from its tampered fruit, sometimes partaking of the whole orchard before realizing who she is dealing with. We think we are presented with so many options when we browse the product aisles, but in reality most stores only offer one kind of skincare product: the dangerous kind. If you just don't see how a world that makes such wonderful things could be bad, let's flip through the pages of a typical beauty magazine together for a moment, shall we?

Look at this stuff. Isn't it neat? Wouldn't you think our collection's complete? Wouldn't you think we're the girls who have everything? The visages are angelic, the scenery divine. Products cloaked in ruby packaging enchant the viewer's eye. A familiar face entices you to give the brand a try. But inside lurks a potion made of placental extract,[1] Teflon,[2] and a token butterfly.

Since that was so fun (I love singing Disney songs with you), now let's stroll arm and arm through a big box beauty store. *C'mon!*

Look at this trove, treasures untold. How many wonders can one cavern hold? Looking around here you think, "Sure, we've got everything." And it's not just chemical products. We've got whozits and whatzits galore. You want thingamabobs? Sephora's got twenty.

---

[1] "Placental extracts, probably with high concentrations of the hormone progesterone and estrogenic chemicals, are sometimes used in cosmetics and hair care products, particularly products marketed to women of color... Research indicates that use of these products in infants and children may also be linked to precocious puberty or early sexual maturation, a risk factor for later life breast cancer." SOURCE: "Hormones in Personal Care Products," Breast Cancer Fund.

[2] "Newly published test results show that a toxic contaminant linked to cancer known as perfluorooctanoic acid (PFOA) was found in anti-aging products from beloved brands Garnier and CoverGirl. PFOA is a contaminant of polytetrafluoroethylene (PTFE), an ingredient used to create a smooth finish on some cookware and personal care products." SOURCE: "New report from Breast Cancer Fund's Campaign for Safe Cosmetics reveals toxic contaminants in L'Oréal Garnier and P&G Cover Girl products," Press Release, The Campaign for Safe Cosmetics, Oct 14, 2015.

But who cares? No big deal. We deserve *more.*

When I inhale the aroma from a newly-opened jar of moisturizer, I want to feel like I'm right there where the flowers are. I want to see, want to smell them blossom. Breathing in all that, what do you call it? Oh—nature. Relying on synthetic chemicals, you don't get too far. Plants are required for distilling, extracting... infusing into a— what's that word again?—*nontoxic* personal care product.

The reason our beauty products are full of dangerous chemicals is because the entire $71 billion industry is regulated by a mere 591 words of legislation written into the Federal Food, Drug, and Cosmetic Act of 1938. Yes, it was *nineteen thirty-eight* when that happened.

Can you imagine your great grandpa trying to write federal code to regulate the ingredients in your makeup bag? He tried his best to ensure it wouldn't contain substances that are "poisonous," "adulterated," or "putrid."[3] But grandpa, poisonous is such a subjective term. What about carcinogenic, endocrine-disruptive, or lethal to unborn children? He didn't think of those. He also didn't think to require anyone to approve new products before they are put on the market, or to mandate that new chemicals be tested for health effects. Just in case that last line didn't hit you the way it should, I repeat it here in operatic falsetto: *no one is testing and approving our beauty products.*[4]

All efforts to update federal regulation of cosmetics have been subverted by the personal care product industry. Did I mention they make $71 billion per year? When it comes to talk about safety, they don't like a lot of blabber. They think discussions about toxins are a

---

[3] You can read the current legislation in United States Code, Title 21, Chapter 9, Subchapter VI, sections 361-364.

[4] When the lack of regulation started to give the cosmetics industry a bad reputation, the industry itself set up a Cosmetics Ingredient Review panel to at least give the appearance of propriety. Out of over ten thousand unique chemicals used in personal care products, the industry panel has declared only 11 ingredients or chemical groups to be unsafe in its 30+ year history. Furthermore, companies are not required to avoid those chemicals in their products. So no, that does not count as regulation. SOURCE: "Myths on cosmetics safety," The Environmental Working Group.

bore. In D.C. it's much preferred for ladies not to say a word. After all dear, what are federal bureaucrats for? Come on, they're not all that impressed with scientific evidence. True gentlemen avoid it when they can. But they dote and swoon and fawn on a scientist who's a pawn. Few chemicals that cause cancer have been banned. (*cymbals!*)

To peddle their poison, they unfortunately know a little magic. It's a marketing talent that they always have possessed. And dear lady, please don't laugh; they use it on behalf of the miserable, the lonely, and depressed. Pathetic.

When your face is covered in breakouts, you'll take desperate measures to feel human again. I was once one of those poor, unfortunate souls. So sad, so true. We go flocking to their cauldrons crying, "Spells, Ulta, please!" And they help us. Yes, they do.

What other option do we have? Either we slather our faces in potentially toxic sludge or hide in our seashells all day. Life's full of tough choices, isn'it?

Well, angelfish, the solution to our problem is simple. The only way to get what you want is to become a cosmetics regulator yourself. "Can you do that?" My dear, sweet child, that's what I do. That's what consumer advocacy groups like the Campaign for Safe Cosmetics and the Environmental Working Group live for—to help unfortunate consumers like ourselves. Poor souls with no one else to turn to. Online resources like SafeCosmetics.org and the Skin Deep Database[5] make it easy to research the potential health effects of the warts, pus, and pig farts allowed to be included in your beauty balm.

But be forewarned. Reading labels doesn't always help. Some of the most noxious chemicals, such as 1,4-dioxane and porcine flatus, won't be listed on the bottle. Since none of the federal agencies are regulating personal care products, there is no one to require companies to put toxic or allergenic ingredients on product labels. Grandpa didn't think of that rule, either. The system he set up to protect us from industry hazards is a complete failure. Sorry grandpa, but it's true.

---

[5] www.ewg.org/skindeep/

We are bright young women, sick of swimming in a sea of questionable cosmetics. Ready to take a stand. Ready to know what the manufacturers know. Ask them our questions and get some answers. Like what's in mascara and why does it, what's the word... *BURN!*

Oh, and there is one more thing. We haven't discussed the subject of payment. You can't get something for nothing, you know. And I'm not just talking about the price tag. There's another small price they ask of you when you purchase a mass-marketed beauty product. It's a token really, a trifle. What they want from you is: your voice.

Every time you purchase a personal care product, you are voicing your support for the retailer, the manufacturer, and the entire regulatory system that enabled the product to be conjured into being. Now it's happened once or twice, someone had to pay an even bigger price, and I'm afraid coal tar is *still* not banned 80+ years later.[6] The beauty industry has had more than the odd complaint. On the whole they've *not* been saints to us poor unfortunate souls.

The long-term solution isn't just to purchase the "natural" line from the same old companies at the same old retail outlets. They might admit that in the past they've been a nasty. (I wasn't kidding when I called them, well, a witch.) But they'll claim that nowadays they've mended all their ways. Repented, seen the light, and made a switch. True? No.

These companies are too big to care about individual tadpoles, even if they wanted to. They have portfolios to maintain, stock holders to appease, and decades of procedure to determine which direction they will swim. They might ride the currents of consumer trends and

---

[6] "In 1933, a woman was hospitalized with excruciating eye pain. Doctors watched in horror as her eyes were eaten away as though by acid. The culprit turned out to be an eyelash-darkening treatment called Lash Lure, which contained paraphenylenediamine, a toxic coal tar dye." SOURCE: Sigurdson, Tina. "Exposing the Cosmetics Cover-Up: True Horror Stories of Cosmetic Dangers," The Environmental Working Group, Oct 29, 2013.

use their mystical marketing powers to take on the appearance of younger companies who genuinely build their brands on the use of pure and organic ingredients, but that does not disguise the fact that they are old outmoded corporations at heart. If you continue purchasing from them, my poor little poopsies, you'll have your looks, your pretty face, but don't underestimate the importance of *fine print legal language.*

So go ahead. Make your choice. If you want to keep on buying the same cosmetics at Macy's, I understand.[7] You're a very busy woman and you haven't got all day to find a replacement for your favorite face cream. It won't cost much. Just your voice. If you want to cross the bridge, my sweet, you've got to pay the toll. Take a gulp and take a breath and go ahead and sell your soul. Johnson & Johnson, now they've got you, girls. The beauty industry's on a roll. You poor, unfortunate soul.

[Intermission]

While you would make a charming addition to the beauty industry's little garden of wayward spirits, you don't need a kiss from a prince, your adopted step-mother, or even your sister to wake up from their spell. If I know you, the waves of doubt are already rising to the forefront of your mind. Maybe a Brazilian Blowout gave you hypotrichosis (Greek caveman for "depressed hair condition," or hair loss), and now you are questioning the concoctions of shampoo on

---

[7] In 2012, the Campaign for Safe Cosmetics ranked Macy's at the bottom of the list of retailers who support the use of safe cosmetics. Macy's does not have a policy to screen for personal care products of concern. Instead, the company has stated that current regulatory standards are adequate for ensuring personal care product safety. Macy's relies on vendors to meet safety standards. SOURCE: "Retailer Therapy," The Campaign for Safe Cosmetics, 2012.

your shower shelf.[8] Maybe you are wondering about your monthly manicure after reading the *New York Times* article about the high incidence of salon workers who have lung diseases, miscarriages, and special-needs children because of their work in the industry.[9]

You might not know why, but you're dying to try—you want to kiss goodbye to conventional beauty products. Well, now's your moment, floating in a blue lagoon of fluorescent chemical fabrications. Boy, you better do it soon. No time will be better.

It might appear as if the big commercial beauty corporations are the rulers of the ocean, that the winds of politics obey their every whim, the sea and all its spoils harnessed for their mass market wares. But you have other options. You won't find them at most national retail chains, but some companies stake their reputations on the integrity of their wizardry. Hand-crafted, wild-harvested, infused with good intentions—these are the kinds of ingredients you will find on their labels. Some retailers too, like Whole Foods, set their own standards about what chemicals they allow in their cupboards.[10]

In 2004, a non-profit group sponsored the Compact for Safe Cosmetics asking manufacturers to sign a pledge to fully disclose ingredients, to avoid the use of chemicals banned in other countries, and to prohibit the use of those linked to cancer or birth defects. By 2011, the campaign listed over 500 manufacturers who satisfied their standards for healthier products.

Zut alors, they have missed one! *Sacre bleu*, what is this? How on earth could they miss such a sweet little succulent beauty product manufacturer. I'm referring to *you*. Homemade beauty products and single-ingredient potions are some of the most luxurious beauty

---

[8] Sigurdson, Tina; Roth, Galen. "Brazilian-Style Blowouts: Still Poisonous, Still In Salons," Environmental Working Group, Aug 21, 2015.

[9] Nir, Sarah Maslin. "Perfect Nails, Poisoned Workers," *The New York Times,* May 8, 2015.

[10] Whole Foods ranked #1 on the Campaign for Safe Cosmetic's list of retailers who support the use of safe personal care products. SOURCE: "Retailer Therapy," The Campaign for Safe Cosmetics, 2012.

treatments in the world. Since I am a simple kind of merwoman, this is the option I often use for myself. For example, diluted raw apple cider vinegar makes for a refreshing toner. And for a moisturizer—some coconut oil, just a dab.[11]

Here's something for tempting the palette, prepared in the classic technique. First you pound some herbs flat with a mallete. Then you slash off their leaves. Give their dry ends a slice. Then you rub sea salt in 'cause it makes it feel nice.

Home beauty treatments are an essential part of the everyday health tradition in many cultures, from the *mandi bunga* flower baths of Malaysia to the famous scented Ayurveda oils of India. *Quel domage,* what a loss we forgot how to make our own sauce.

But not all of us have forgotten, or if we did, we are now starting to remember. Relying on little more than their kitchen sinks, kitchen counters, and kitchen gardens, a new cadre of modern sorceress has taken root throughout the country as they experiment with the lost art of beauty alchemy. They are hybrid creatures, half mortal, half evolved breed of beauty product manufacturer unlike those found in stores.

I met one such phoenix online while blogging at The Cellulite Investigation. Maggie's degree is in architecture from Harvard's Graduate School of Design, but now she works as a mixer of potions, evoking the scents of her native Persia from her West Hollywood kitchen. Her company, Lalun Naturals, is named after a village in the Alborz mountains of Iran where she picnicked under a walnut tree with her family as a child.

Ordering a potion from Maggie is like having your own personalized apothecary. A magical one, of course. She sells a skincare line that changes with the seasons—lavender in summer, calendula in fall, rosehips in winter, and orange blossoms in spring. Maggie's creations are so exclusive they aren't sold in stores, but they are readily

---

[11] For more info on the products I use, see **ProjectFree.Me/Skincare**.

available to those who seek them on her website and on Etsy.[12]

In fact, Etsy is filled with personal care products from magicians like Maggie. Reminiscing just now about the scent of her inspired winter rose moisturizer made from rosehip seed, raw shea butter, and macadamia oil, I had a vision of what the world would look like if more people knew they could buy exquisite personal care products from micro-companies like Maggie's. That world has fewer synthetic chemicals, fewer side effects. More gardens, more Maggies. Instead of waiting to start gardening in retirement, more people are able to follow their natural passion for plants and flowers, working out of their homes creating herbal works of art.

Internet proposes that artists like Maggie don't need their creations to go viral to be successful. It is possible they could make a healthy living with a modest number of devotees.[13] The story of industrialization (and Cinderella) would lead us to believe that companies that start in basements need to end up in corporate castles to be considered a success. But what if instead of going to the ball, Cinderella stayed home and read *The 4-Hour Workweek* by Tim Ferris and then set up her own small business selling natural cleansers, lotions, and other beauty products online? Might she have freed herself from her evil step-mother and lived out her days singing show tunes to adoring forest creatures while foraging for wild herbs with Jaq and Gus-Gus? They would have been so good at that. Who knows, maybe her happily ever after would have been even happier.

Looking around at our present situation, I know my vision for a beauty industry composed of an independent network of Glinda the Good Witches seems like a fairy tale.[14] But we buy into the current model with every lotion we purchase. What if we bought into the fairy tale model instead?

---

[12] www.lalunnaturals.com

[13] See "1,000 True Fans" by Kevin Kelly, the founding executive editor of *Wired* magazine (available at kk.org/thetechnium/1000-true-fans/).

[14] Why do I picture them all flying around in pink Cadillacs?

What would I give to live in a world without triclosan? What would I pay to keep you away from BHA? What would I do just to see you, smiling at me with lead-free lipstick? Wandering free, wish we could be part of that world.

When's it our turn? Wouldn't I love not to gauge our beauty products by what they're free of...

[Finale]

Now that we know acne-free skin does not require the use of special skincare products, our facial potions—like all fine works of art —are free to exist purely for the pleasure that comes with indulging our senses in the sweet scents and textures of the natural world, with the added bonus of providing a little extra luminescence when desired.

A better beauty industry already exists; we don't need to wait for government princes to take us there. The alchemists who create such masterpieces are already among us, we just need to find and support them until we reach the tipping point and their good magic spreads throughout the land. I know it won't happen overnight, but if you believe in fairytale endings, I will believe in them too. Now, do we have a deal?

If you haven't done so already, you can start to enter this new world by choosing just one type of personal care product in your repertoire and finding a version that supports our shared vision for what the beauty industry should look like.[15] It doesn't have to be a Maggie. Just find a source that defines itself on the use of nothing but quality ingredients, and then try to purchase it through a retailer who takes care not to poison masses of people with their products.

The key is not to put it off. Choose a product from your bathroom shelf *right now*. We mustn't lurk in doorways, it's rude.

---

[15] For some suggestions to get you started, see **ProjectFree.Me/Skincare**.

[Reprise]

I don't know when. I don't know how. But I know something's starting right now. Watch and you'll see. Someday we'll be part of *that* world.

*****

Your Inner Mermaid Visits Oz

To understand which skincare treatments are the most effective at healing breakouts, we need to revisit an unanswered question that arose in Part One of our story. What exactly is going on inside our bodies that causes the fluoride we eat and drink to end up on our faces? I have a theory, but it requires us to try to view the human body with fresh eyes. Here is a story designed to help us do just that.

In *The Little Mermaid* when Ariel has a question about "human stuff," she ventures to the surface to ask her seagull friend, Scuttle. Let's say for the purpose of this exercise that one day, perhaps not long after the time she rescues Eric from drowning but before her bargain with Ursula, Ariel starts wondering about the physiology of humans that allows them to live outside of the water. When she arrives at Scuttle's place, he just so happens to be having lunch with America's favorite doctor, Mehmet Oz. A lively conversation ensues.

"Whoa! Mermaid off the port bow!" Scuttle says as he greets Ariel at his buoy door. Pointing at Dr. Oz, he warns her under his breath, "Look at what the catfish dragged in." You see, Mehmet had gotten into the habit of dropping by in the afternoons without notice, and it was starting to interfere with Scuttle's snarfblatt practice. After a quick introduction and a few pleasantries, Ariel begins asking her questions about human physiology.

When the conversation turns to matters of the human body, Dr. Oz's face lights up like a little mergirl in a dinglehopper shop. He quickly whips out an autographed copy of his bestselling health book, entitled *You: The Owner's Manual*. Flipping to the table of contents, he explains that each chapter covers a major system of the human body. You've got the heart and veins, the brain, the musculoskeletal system, the lungs, the gut, the sexual organs, the sensory organs, the immune system, and the hormonal system.

Ariel tries to listen politely to Dr. Oz's enthusiastic explanation of C-reactive protein, but she can't keep her mind from wandering back to her mermaid anatomy class in high school. Mermaids have hearts and brains and muscles and bones. Like their closest ocean relative, the dolphin, they even have lungs. But why is it that if she tried to live with Eric on land she would soon shrivel and die like a beached whale?

What was so special about humans that they could stay all day in the sun? Jumping, dancing, strolling around on those—what do you call them? Oh wait, this isn't a musical scene. Sorry.

Ariel interrupts the doc just as he was getting to the good part about homocysteine and arterial inflammation. "But how do they live outside of the ocean?!" she demands.

Sensing Ariel was losing her patience, Scuttle jumps in with an explanation. "Out of the ocean? Oh... uh, yes. Excellent question." He clears his throat, "In prehysterical times when humans first decided to live out of the ocean, they just took the ocean with 'em."

Scuttle then grabs Dr. Oz by both ears and stares deeply at his forehead. "Yep, there it is," he states, matter-of-fact. "I can see it leaking out of his thick water-balloon skull right now."

Without looking away from Oz's face, Scuttle reaches down and grabs the napkin from under his dinglehopper. He then presses it against Dr. Oz's brow which at this point was sweating quite profusely due to the noonday sun reflecting off the water and the pressure of such a heated line of questioning from a fiery red-headed mermaid.

Scuttle then wrings the napkin over a young crop of seaweed growing in a bulbous snarfblatt nearby. "You see?" he says triumphantly. "Saltwater."

Not wanting to be shown up by a know-it-all seagull, Dr. Oz tries to recompose himself by resorting to an old doctor's tactic (you probably saw this one before) where he throws out a statistic to demonstrate his expertise on a topic. "Actually, Scuttle is onto something here," Dr. Oz says as he runs his hands through his hair in an attempt to reshape it back into an aesthetically pleasing configuration. "About two thirds of the human body is water."

Ariel raises an auburn eyebrow in suspicion. "If the human body is mostly water, then why isn't *water* one of the chapters in your book?" she asks.

Dr. Oz thinks for a moment. "Well, I... I suppose it could have been in there, but...you know, we had a limited number of pages and..."

Not willing to let this one go, Ariel continues to press him on the matter. "In fact, if the human body is mostly water, shouldn't it be the very first chapter?" she asks him. Realizing Oz is finally at a loss for words, she instinctively turns to chapter one in search of an answer to her own question.

"Look!" she says, pointing at the page in excitement. "Right here on page three you say: 'your heart is your water main.' How poetic!"

Ariel sighs and hugs the book to her chest before asking, "In the human body, is the heart beating water?"

Dr. Oz shakes his head. This is not going at all like the conversations he has with human women on television. "That was just an analogy," he explains. "The heart pumps *blood* through the body, providing nutrients for all the organs and tissues. It's the most life-giving organ we have which is why I wrote about it first. It's why people write poems about it and use its image to decorate candy boxes, boxer shorts, and Valentine's day cards."

(Ariel didn't ask this next question out loud because, to be honest, she was growing tired of the doctor's answers and didn't want to set him off on another tangent. But she wondered to herself, "If blood is what is actually providing the nutrients for their bodies, then why don't humans decorate their Valentine's day cards with blood instead of abstract symbols that don't even look like real hearts? She thought it was a very clever idea and decided she would try it next February on her card for Eric.)

When Ariel looked up from her book, Scuttle's guest had moved on from waxing poetic about aortic valves and was now talking about clogs and clots and other trouble spots. He was just making his way back to the good part about homocysteine when Ariel thought up an excuse about missing a concert for her father and swam off into the fathoms below.

*****

I hope that by submerging yourself in Ariel's point of view, this silly story is helping you see the human body at least a little differently. We tend to fixate so intensely on our modern interpretations that we forget they are only a story of the world and not the world itself.

In western medicine, we focus on organs that we can hold in our hands or feel beating under our chest. We try to name everything and define it by how it is different from everything else. But there are other interpretations of the human body that are just as valid, just as descriptive. To give an example, let's see what conclusion Ariel reaches regarding her curiosity about what it would take to leave the ocean and become human (physiologically speaking, for now).

Impressed by Dr. Oz's statistic about the human body being composed primarily of water, Ariel returns to the secret cave where she stores all her human treasures and pores over every page of his book until something catches her eye. She notices several passing references to drains, often in connection with a mysterious system referred to as "lymphatic." Intrigued, she does what any smart modern mermaid would do. She looks it up on Merkipedia.

Ariel reads the first sentence to Flounder out loud, "The lymphatic system is part of the circulatory system and a vital part of the immune system, comprising a network of lymphatic vessels that carry a clear fluid called lymph (from Latin *lympha,* meaning water) directionally towards the heart."

"Water," she whispers with hushed excitement. "That's it, Flounder. We found it! We found the ocean inside the human body!"

Ariel learns that lymph, like sweat and tears, is basically a type of saltwater. The human body contains twice as much lymph as it does blood, which makes her wonder why Oz went on and on (and on) about the cardiovascular system but didn't think to mention the liters of saltwater circulating through his body at that very moment.

In his book, *You: The Owner's Manual,* Dr. Oz explains the lymphatic system briefly as a side note in his chapter on immunity, right below his descriptions of the thymus, bone marrow, spleen, and the baby hairs that develop on human pinky toes. According to Oz, the lymphatic system is a series of nodes where immune activity takes place, with the nodes acting as filters that move waste from infections out of the body. He doesn't even acknowledge the existence of lymph or the extensive system of lymphatic vessels that extend to every organ and tissue.

Ariel then checks out Dr. Oz's blog where he describes the lymphatic system a little differently. Flounder laughs his tail fin off as she musters her best Oz impersonation to read the description aloud. She begins eyes wide, hands posed for gesticulation with her fingers outstretched as if she just slid them into a pair of latex gloves.[16]

"Imagine your body is a house," she says while outlining the crude shape of a house with her hands. "Fresh water is kept under a

---

[16] Like this: www.nbc.com/saturday-night-live/video/ask-dr-oz/n13252.

certain amount of pressure in an intricate system of pipes in order for it to circulate around the house." Ariel pauses to find a shipwrecked toilet seat to use as a visual aid. "Your house has another system of pipes, drainpipes, which take used water out of the house to the sewer system or septic tank, so your house doesn't flood with water." She is sitting on the toilet seat now as she reads this last line, "Your lymphatic system is *that* system of drainpipes."

"Gross!" Flounder interjects. "Lymph is like dirty toilet water?"

"No, that's just an analogy," Ariel explains. "He's not always good with analogies."

The lymphatic system has long been overshadowed by the more colorful blood circulatory system because it doesn't have a flamboyant character like the heart to help circulate lymph around the body. Also, most lymph vessels are difficult to see even upon dissection. In western medicine, the lymphatic system wasn't even discovered until the seventeenth century when some guys in Sweden and Denmark who no one cares about anymore anyway started fighting over who noticed it first. Lymph had already been incorporated into eastern medicine for centuries where the idea of lymph was bound up in conceptions of "*qi*" or "*prana,*" or it was expressed simply as "damp."

This latter depiction provides an insightful way of viewing extracellular fluid, our word for the fluid that exists outside our cells. Our term lymph is limited to fluid that is contained inside lymphatic vessels. But before this fluid enters the lymphatic vessels, it is considered interstitial fluid—the fluid that bathes our cells. The defining characteristic between interstitial fluid and lymphatic fluid is location. But no matter where it is located in the body, isn't it all just saltwater?

In western medicine, we choose to define these internal fluids by their placement in the human body. That is our script and we follow it. But trying to explain the inner workings of the human body with words is like trying to hold a moonbeam in your hand from twenty thousand leagues under the sea. We can tell stories about nature, but our stories will never capture its full being.

Dr. Oz might think of lymph as dirty toilet water, but perhaps an inquisitive mermaid would find it more akin to the ever-present experience of *ocean*. (And then she would sing a lively song about it with a Rastafarian crab who I did not include in this story because we had limited time for character development. However, if you listen attentively through the remainder of this chapter, at the end I promise to share with you the song they sing together. It's very catchy.)

Now that Ariel's line of inquiry has revealed the inner ocean which bathes every cell in the human body, we can more easily see how the fluoride we consume through our diet ends up on our faces. When our bodies are already full of fluoride and then we consume food and beverages with more fluoride, some of it makes its way into our lymphatic circulation and can cause congestion in our body's fluids. That is why when you are overloaded with fluoride, your sweat smells different, your breath stinks, your tongue might turn white, and your skin desperately attempts to bail itself out by erupting in a clear liquid it tries to throw overboard. If you pay close attention to the pattern of your breakouts, you might even be able to trace some of the pathways of the lymphatic vessels that drain lymph towards your heart.

When the waters of your inner ocean start to stagnate from over-pollution, there are many steps you can take to help them flow freely again. Now that you know my theory that fluoride causes acne by congesting your lymphatic system, it should be clear that any activity that improves lymphatic circulation will help to prevent and heal breakouts. As Ariel's conversation with Oz demonstrates, the lymphatic system doesn't have a pump to help circulate lymph throughout the body. Instead, it relies on a type of peristalsis that is stimulated by a combination of skeletal movement and pressure changes in the chest cavity during breathing. In other words, lymph flows as a function of movement and breath.

For many Americans, there are two kinds of exercise: weight training and cardio. Notice they both focus on working your muscles. If your heart muscle is pounding at the recommended beat per minute, then you are maximizing your workout. But if we designed our exercises with the lymphatic system in mind, they would look a lot different.

Instead of focusing exclusively on muscles, we would focus on stimulating lymphatic flow by leveraging movement with breath. We would probably move into certain positions we don't commonly use in daily life, and then take a deep breath to encourage that angle of lymphatic circulation. If we really wanted to shake lymph up, we would incorporate some movements that reverse the regular pull of gravity—you know, turn the lava lamp upside down and let the bubbles float to the top for a minute or two. To be acutely aware of our inner waterworld, we would spend centuries carefully observing the effects of breath on various poses, perhaps even developing complex breathing exercises to influence the tides and currents of the ocean within. Instead, we are still trying to run faster, farther, and longer. Will we ever get there?

The lymphatic system is widely neglected in conventional approaches to health in the United States, but it's a different story in other parts of the world. While Americans focus on working their muscles, the exercise traditions in Asia are centered on movement and breath. Practices like yoga, tai chi, and qigong are ideal for improving lymphatic flow and consequently, the health of your skin.

In Europe, the lymphatic system is addressed through manual techniques where the skin is manipulated in a form of massage designed to enhance the circulation of lymphatic fluid. The most popular technique was developed by Emil and Estrid Vodder, two Danish physicians working in the south of France in the 1930s. It is now commonly used in European hospitals where it is prescribed by physicians and even reimbursed by insurance. Acne was one of the conditions the Vodders first treated with their lymph drainage technique. As I mentioned in chapter one, I experienced relief from my cystic acne after a single session of a similar lymph drainage therapy developed by French physician Dr. Bruno Chikly.

Yoga and massage might not be your typical skincare treatments, but I hope it is now apparent why they are more effective at healing acne than virtually any product you will find at...

Oh no. Stop everything. Was that a flash of disappointment I saw in your eyes just now? Don't tell me you're disappointed. I can't take it. You want to slather scented stuff on your face, don't you. You want to glob it on, rub it in and soak in it like Miss Piggy in a fancy French mud bath. You want to put product on your skin *right now* to fix those appalling, painful pustules on your otherwise pretty face.[17]

Well, my friend, you don't think I would let you sink away discontented, did you? Now that you mention it, there are a few rituals you can perform in front of your bathroom mirror to banish existing breakouts on this very night. But be forewarned, you might need to gather some courage to attempt them.

Mirror, mirror, on the wall. Who's the bravest of us all?

*****

From Beauty to the Beast and Back

It's a tale as old as time. Humanity spends millennia painstakingly uncovering a hidden treasure of the natural world, then industrialization steps in and mutates it to the point doctors convince us we don't want it anymore and should do drugs instead.

While modern chemists frantically stir their cauldrons looking for the latest/greatest chemical ingredients to include in their so-called beauty products, the most effective skincare products were discovered

---

[17] Shut up. You're pretty.

ages ago. Some of them we've forgotten, but others have been vilified to the point you might cringe in fear at their very suggestion. But fear not. We already know how the story ends. [Spoiler alert: the Beast is Prince Charming in disguise.]

Though few of us realize it, the most effective skincare product for acne is as plain as the nose on your face. Or to be more precise, it is as plain as the *oil* on the nose on your face. Thousands of years before soap came into widespread usage, people cleansed their skin with oil.

When your inflamed skin is already shining with "excess" oil, it might feel scary to put more oil on your face, but that's your dermatologist's story—the one where your acne-prone skin is caused by your crazy hormones and your over-productive oil glands. In our story, your acne-prone skin is caused by your crazy dentist and your over-polluted lymphatic system. Oil is the body's way of handling that congestion by sending extra fluid out through the pores. Cleansing your face with oil augments this natural process by helping dissolve fat-soluble substances on your skin.

Dermatologists might have succeeded in convincing us that cleansing oily skin with oil is a ludicrous idea, but chemists, nature, ancient Romans, and popular health bloggers like Mommypotamus tell us otherwise.

In chemistry, the term lipophilicity is Greek caveman for *lipid-loving*. It refers to the ability of a chemical compound to dissolve in fats and oils. Over the years, chemists noticed that lipid-loving substances tend to dissolve in other lipid-loving substances. It is an axiom referred to as "like dissolves like." Water-loving (i.e., *hydro*philic) substances dissolve in other water-loving substances, but to dissolve the oil on your face you will need another oil. This axiom of lipophilicity explains why bathers in the famous baths of ancient Rome cleansed their skin by rubbing oil into their bodies and then scraping it off using a curved metal tool called a *strigil*.

Traditional oils like olive and coconut have a long history of use for skincare in many cultures. But if oil is so great at cleansing oily skin, then why does it have such a bad reputation for clogging pores? That's a good story. How about we let Matthew McConaughey tell it.

After growing up in non-fluoridated Uvalde, Texas, Matthew moved to fluoridated Longview, Texas prior to high school where he developed a severe case of acne. His mom was selling cosmetics door-to-door and suggested he try a product she was peddling, oil of mink. (To say it like Matthew, you need some extra drawl on the word oil. Like this: "oooooooil of mink." Good.)

McConaughey tells the rest of the story to Jimmy Fallon on *The Tonight Show*, "So I start doing the mink oil masks at night, and my face is starting to swell up, and I'm developing really bad acne. I talked to my dad's secretary, who turned my mom onto it. I'm really concerned. And the lady's like, 'Wow, you just sure have a lot of impurities, Matthew. Keep it up! And we'll just pull all of the impurities out, and you'll never have a blemish again.'"

The story ends with Matthew at the dermatologist's office who predictably chides him to stop putting oil on his already oily face and instead gives him a bottle of Inflammatory Bowel Disease (i.e., acne medication). His mother sues the manufacturer of her mink oil product for $30,000 but loses when the judge is shown a photograph that proves Matthew was still voted Most Handsome in his high school class.

Looking at Matthew McConaughey's acne story, it is not that different than the tale dentists tell about fluoridation. His mom, his dad's secretary, and teenaged Matthew himself are the helpless and confused townspeople. The dermatologist is the wise hero. Industrial poison is the magic potion the hero uses to save the day. The judge is the government official who sides with industry lawyers because of a distracting but irrelevant picture of a smiling child with sparkly white teeth.

If we didn't know better, stories like Matthew's seem to confirm the idea that oil causes acne. But just like in the story of fluoridation, there is an industry chemist and a few admen trying their best to hide behind a cardboard cactus on the back of the stage.

What is this mysterious "oil of mink" the big bad beauty industry was marketing to women and our future leading men in the 1980s? We find some insights into this question in a 1994 document (thank you, Internet) written by economics professor DeeVon Bailey at the University of Utah in which he outlines his diabolical plot for Utah to take over the mink oil manufacturing world.[18] Or at least the coveted *cosmetics* mink oil manufacturing world. Or maybe just the leather care market. Or perhaps they could sell it to local shoe stores? Or they could create their own shoe stores and then sell it to them? Anyway.

The document explains that most mink oil in Utah is marketed as a low grade oil used primarily to feed factory-farmed livestock. Dr. Bailey's plot suggests that if Utah manufacturers adopted a fractional distillation process like those savvy mink companies in Wisconsin, then Utah mink oil might live a life of luxury in high end beauty lotions or leather coats instead of ending up as cow caca. Bailey cites Avon and Kiwi as two companies that use "highly processed" mink oil in their product lines. He explains that cosmetics companies use mink oil in skincare products like creams and lotions, while leather care companies use it to treat, preserve, and waterproof leather.

Now, I'm not a beauty product manufacturer *or* a leather specialist, so I am doubly forced to rely on my little layman brain for this one, but if a product is able to keep fluids out, might it also have the effect of keeping fluids in? Even when those fluids are bodily fluids that aren't supposed to stay in? It makes sense why Mother Nature would use a water-proofing oil for a semiaquatic animal like mink, but as Mathew McConaughey selflessly tried to show us, waterproofing a human face might not be the best option for healing acne.

Ooooil of mink might sound luxurious, especially the way

---

[18] Bailey, DeeVon; Thomsen, Michael R., "An Initial Analysis of the Mink Oil Market: Preliminary Report to Morgan County, Utah," Utah State University, Jan 19, 1994.

Matthew McConaughey says it, but it is not a traditional oil for skincare. As Dr. Bailey and his minions demonstrate, the use of mink oil in cosmetics is more an attempt by the fur industry to increase revenue by selling a byproduct of imprisoned minks as something other than cheap fodder for imprisoned cows.

Dermatologists fail to differentiate this type of heavily processed industrialized oil from more traditional oils used for skincare when deciphering oil's role in the causes and cures for acne. While adolescent Matthew was slathering his future Oscar-winning face with mutated mink oil in the 1980s, people started noticing similar side effects from other industrialized cosmetic oils. In an attempt to throw consumers off their trail, industry marketers created a secret beauty product language consisting of words like *"hypo-allergenic,"* *"non-comedogenic,"* and *"dermatologist-approved."* Consumers assumed these new words meant someone was looking out for the safety of their beauty products and that potions inscribed with such symbols would not clog pores. But in legal terms, these are nonsense words, the way "wiggle" is the color of pink lipstick.

Because of the mass confusion over the role of oil in the cause of acne, it was widely banished as a modern skincare cleanser in the latter half of the twentieth century. It remained locked away in a castle tower until Internet revived interest in it with a mysterious little website called TheOilCleansingMethod.com.

The site was created by Stephanie Strauss, a stay-at-home mom who in the early 1990s read a book that recommended cleansing your face with olive oil. The idea intrigued her so she tried it and immediately fell in love with the soft, supple skin that resulted. She was also intrigued by a new toy called the World Wide Web and created a simple website to tell people about cleansing with oil. It was just a few pages, but after 15 years online it managed to attract the attention of some of the most popular natural health and beauty bloggers, such as Mommypotamus,[19] Crunchy Betty,[20] and Wellness Mama (<3).[21]

Just like thousands of other American women in her demographic, Stephanie has adult acne and is prone to breakouts along her chin and jawline. She suggests using a castor oil blend to cleanse your face, but she also recommends mineral oil and the occasional light soaping with Johnson & Johnson's baby wash—two highly-industrialized chemical products that show she has not yet fully awoken from the industry's spell.

You don't need to use a particular blend to cleanse your skin with oil. Castor oil is widely recommended because of Stephanie's site, but it is a potent medicinal oil that can cause strong reactions—it is made from the same plant used to produce ricin. Traditional skincare oils are nourishing in different ways, so you might have to experiment with a few oils to find the ones you like best. Jojoba, coconut, olive, and almond oil are some of the most versatile. Or you could consult a beauty mystic like Maggie who formulates her oil cleansers to balance with the seasons, extra hydrating in winter and more absorbent in summer months.

The way oils are grown and processed can also influence how they affect your face. Maggie only uses organic oils that are extracted using traditional cold pressed methods. If your skin does not react well to a certain oil, remember the hard-earned lesson we learned from Matthew McConaughey: stop using it and try something else.

You don't need detailed instructions for oil cleansing, either. The premise is simple. Massage a traditional oil used in skincare into your skin (as opposed to a highly processed industrialized oil used in mink enslavement, *Matthew!*). Then gently remove it. You can start with wet skin or dry skin. You can use circular motions or upward

---

[19] www.mommypotamus.com/oil-cleansing-for-clear-baby-soft-skin-video-tutorial/

[20] www.crunchybetty.com/nitty-gritty-on-the-oil-cleansing-method

[21] www.wellnessmama.com/7569/oil-cleansing-method/

strokes. You can massage for 30 seconds or 2 minutes. You can remove the oil with a warm washcloth, a cold washcloth, a tissue, a cotton round, a pot holder, a Matthew McConaughey t-shirt, a doily, or your dog's tongue. (Just kidding, I don't do that. Seriously, I don't.)

My favorite method for removing oil from my skin is a strigil-like tool similar to what the ancient Roman's used to scrape off oil and dead skin cells. I found it at a discount store several years ago. It was originally sold by QVC but is no longer on the market. A company created a similar product called LeEdge, but that seems to be out of production now too, replaced by a new product which I have not yet tried called Exfolimate. Clearly the market for Roman strigils is experiencing a moment of volatility but I will try to keep you updated with the latest options at **ProjectFree.Me/Skincare**.

While strigil-like tools are the best facial exfoliators I know of, their utility is limited if you have active breakouts because they can only be used on smooth skin. But there is another tool that has a longstanding tradition of use in conjunction with oils, and it is even more effective at improving lymphatic circulation.

Next to acupuncture, cupping therapy is the primary technique used in Traditional Chinese Medicine to reduce stagnation in qi and internal fluids. It was also practiced by early Egyptians before it spread to ancient Greece and many countries in Europe and even the Americas. In cupping therapy, cups are used to create suction against the skin, pulling the tissue upward like an inverse massage. The earliest references to cupping involved the use of animal horns and then jars made of bamboo or pottery. Glass cups eventually came into widespread use, but now silicone cups are readily available and make it easy to incorporate this ancient practice into your home skincare routine.

A gentle type of cupping called "glide cupping" is the treatment I relied on when I needed to heal a breakout quickly. I found it can even prevent a blemish from surfacing if I treated it early enough. Instructions for glide cupping are simple. After massaging your face with oil, squeeze the cup to create a light suction and then release it against your skin. Lymph capillaries are sensitive, so you only need to use enough suction to keep the cup attached. Then glide the cup across your face. You don't need to run the cup directly over the breakout for cupping to be effective. Doing so could aggravate already tender skin. Instead, focus on improving the overall flow of lymph. I like to start at my neck with several downward strokes before moving to the problem area on my chin and around the sides of my mouth. I'll also incorporate some long strokes along my jawline towards my ears and from the inside edge of my eyebrow across my forehead. The idea is to move in the general direction of lymphatic flow.[22]

In Stephanie's oil cleansing method, she recommends draping a hot towel over your face, "essentially steaming [y]our skin as an esthetician would, but without the luxury of a steam machine." A hot towel feels nice, but you also could have the luxury of a steam machine for about the same price as the Egyptian cotton washcloths Stephanie recommends on her site. Small facial saunas start at as little as twenty dollars and can work your skin into a healthy sweat in less than ten minutes. I found them to be much more effective than leaning over a bowl of hot water. Steaming your face won't prevent acne if you are still consuming fluoride, but it is an excellent treatment for those occasions when you accidentally consume some fluoridated California wine out of a dancing punchbowl, for example, and have a few breakouts you want to heal before an important date with a bewitched prince.

Depending on your powers of perception, you might have noticed at some point over the years that the skin on your face is connected to the rest of your body. While facial saunas are a great option if you are tight on money or space, they can't compare to the health benefits of a full body version. From the sweat lodges of

---

[22] For a video demonstration and more information on cupping to heal acne, visit ProjectFree.me/Facial-Cupping-Video.

Mesoamerica to the weekly sauna rituals in northern Europe and the hammams of the Muslim world, saunas are a longstanding tradition in many cultures for improving skin health and general detoxification. It is a shame they have been largely abandoned in modern American life.

I did my part to bring back saunas after reading *Sauna Therapy for Detoxification and Healing* by Lawrence Wilson. At first, I used a far-infrared sauna purchased from a friend when she moved overseas. But eventually, I upgraded to a near-infrared sauna like Dr. Wilson recommends in his book. Near-infrared saunas are about the price of a MacBook, or you can build one yourself for under two hundred dollars. If you live in a fluoridated house and don't want to take baths in industrial pollution, they are the perfect alternative for 30 minutes of luxury me-time. Every home should have one. If the Finns can do it, why can't we? (For more information on saunas and other tools discussed in this chapter, see **ProjectFree.Me/Skincare**.)

Let's see. We talked about cleansing your face with oil. We talked about increasing sweat. What other traditional skincare solutions have been neglected in recent years? Oh right, dirt.

One of the most effective remedies for healing breakouts quickly is dirt, or more specifically, clay. The first recorded use of medicinal clay was in ancient Mesopotamia, but some scholars (and Wikipedia) believe clay was used to heal wounds even in prehistoric times. Ancient Egyptians, Classical Romans, Medieval Persians, Renaissance Europeans, and Crunchy Californians all used clay as a traditional healing compound.

The term *"bentonite"* refers to a variety of absorbent clays derived from volcanic ash. There are a lot of scientific explanations for why bentonite clay is helpful in healing acne, but I didn't read any of them when I first started using it. I based my decision solely on the 6,000+ reviewers who rave about bentonite clay on Amazon. A 1-pound canister costs less than eight dollars.

You can get super fancy with clay, but I followed the directions on the label and mixed a spoonful with equal parts organic apple cider vinegar and water. It whips into a delightful green froth that feels like marshmallow cream when first applied, but soon hardens your face into Venus de Milo. After just 20 minutes, my breakouts were well on their way to being ancient history. It was magic.

Or science. Same diff. Bentonite clay is scientifically proven to be exceedingly good at absorbing human sebum. In fact, when scientists conduct studies on how much sebum is secreted by humans, they sometimes use bentonite clay to measure it. It's a technique they affectionately refer to as the bentonite method.[23]

Another science-y reason bentonite clay is especially good at healing breakouts is because it carries a strong negative charge which is said to bond with the positive charge in many toxins. The toxins I've seen don't have their electrical charges listed on the ingredient label (*of course*), but I found NWCag's YouTube video to be compelling evidence that this line of reasoning is worth further investigation.[24] In the video, he connects two wires to the positive and negative charges on a battery, and then places the other end of each wire into a beaker of bentonite clay mixed with water. When he removes the wires from the clay, the negatively charged wire comes out clean but because opposite charges attract, the positively charged wire is covered in a clump of clay. Is that not the wildest YouTube video you've ever heard of?

There could be some video editing sleight-of-hand going on here, but NWCag doesn't seem like that kind of guy. He seems like the kind of guy who is affiliated with the agricultural program at Northwest College in Powell, Wyoming and likes to post videos online about geology exercises (32 views), fertilizer calculations (152 views), and soil bulk density (2,180 views—*go Trappers!*).[25]

---

[23] For example, see Downing, D.T.; Stranieri, A.M.; Strauss, J.S. "The effect of accumulated lipids on measurements of sebum secretion in human skin," *The Journal of Investigative Dermatology*, vol. 79, issue 4, 1982, pp. 226-228.

[24] To view the video, see ProjectFree.Me/Bentonite-Clay.

[25] Given the electrical charge of bentonite clay, it is advised that metal not be used when mixing the ingredients of your clay mask. I admit I don't fully understand why, but I use a glass dish and a plastic spoon to make up for my lack of woo insight.

Now feels like a good time to remind you that you don't need to use any of these treatments to maintain clear skin. If you heal your acne by avoiding fluoride, there won't be any breakouts to treat. Once I learned how to eliminate excess fluoride from my diet, clear skin became effortless.

My current skincare routine is a variation of the "caveman regimen" featured on The Love Vitamin, a website created by Tracy Raftl to help women heal their acne naturally. It involves not washing or using any products on your face *at all*.[26] I did not intentionally decide to do this method of skincare, rather I happened into it a few months ago when I temporarily moved to a fluoridated neighborhood. At first, I took the time to wash my face with spring water but now that I'm writing this book, I spend every moment of my free time with you (totally worth it). Superfluous activities like face washing have fallen to the wayside, along with makeup applying, hair doing, jewelry wearing, shoe shopping, and a few other borderline nonessential activities I prefer not to mention. Like eyebrow tweezing. (Melissa, *just stop.*)

Every few days, I use a strigil-like tool in the shower to exfoliate my face. Since my skin is already soft from the shower, I don't even need to apply oil beforehand although I do rub a few drops in afterwards. Other than that, my skin is completely free to do its own thing. I miss my saunas and clay masks because they feel good and make my skin glow, but this conversation with you is so much more important than that.

So there you have it. The skincare products I relied on to heal breakouts fast are: dirt, sweat, and oil. Oh, and a cup. How ironic is it that the primary villains in dermatologists' story of acne ended up being the solution they've been looking for all along? Who would have guessed, right?!

---

[26] Raftl, Tracy. "Am I Still Doing the Caveman Regimen? (Three & a Half Years Later)," Nov 5, 2015 (available at http://thelovevitamin.com/17857/am-i-still-doing-the-caveman-regimen/).

I mean, other than people who write Disney movies. And people who watch Disney movies. And all of antiquity. And the Big 4 Moms: Mother Nature, Mrs. McConaughey, Mrs. Potts, and Mommypotamus.[27]

---

[27] Visit **ProjectFree.Me/Breakouts** to receive a 1-page Quick Guide on how to heal breakouts overnight.

Under the Skin[28]

Seaweed mask is always greener
On somebody else's face
You see doc to make skin clearer
But that is a risky place
Just look at the world around you
Right here in the human pore
Such wonderful things swim 'round you
What more is you lookin' for?

Under the skin
Under the skin
Darling it's better
Be a trendsetter
Oil that grin
There at the doc's they make you pay
To pop the pills (don't work anyway)
While lymph devotin'
Full time to floatin'
Under the skin

Down here all the lymph is happy
They swim, they are never bored
The lymph at the doc's ain't happy
They sad 'cause they is ignored
But lymph that's ignored is lucky
They in for a worser fate
One day when the pills get yucky
Guess who gon' feel des-o-late

[28] Lyric Challenge: Free *Under the Skin* t-shirt for the first person to successfully adapt the following lyrics to an appropriate lymph-loving sentiment. "The newt play the flute, the carp play the harp, the plaice play the bass, and they soundin' sharp. The bass play the brass, the chub play the tub, the fluke is the duke of soul (yeah). The ray he can play, the lings on the strings, the trout rockin' out, the blackfish she sings, the smelt and the sprat, they know where it's at, an' oh that blowfish blow."

Under the skin
Under the skin
Nobody bug us
Charge us and drug us
Gimme some fin
We what the doctor love to lance
Under the skin lymph love to dance
We got no troubles
Lymph flow like bubbles
Under the skin

Under the skin
Under the skin
When the whitehead
Begin to turn red
Lymph fixes my chin
What do they got? A lot of creams
We got the big ocean of our dreams
Each little zit here
Know when to quit here
Under the skin
Each little pimple
Lymph make it simple
Under the skin
All of that acne
It don't attack me
Lymph flow like lava
Only it's hotter
Ya we in luck here
Down in the muck here
Under the skin

6

BECOMING ACNE-PROOF

*"You are braver than you believe,
stronger than you seem,
and smarter than you think."*

—Christopher Robin

THERE IS ONE MORE SOURCE OF FLUORIDE YOU ARE EXPOSED TO that we did not discuss yet. It is the least understood but the most important. As you will soon see, it explains one of the fundamental mysteries of a little phenomenon we refer to as human civilization, amongst other stuff. I didn't include it in chapter four because it's not a source of fluoride you can avoid. You are exposed to it every day. All day. Even while you sleep. There is no getting away from it. Like the great poet Beyonce says, nobody frees you from your body.

If you grew up consuming the typical industrialized diet—drinking fluoridated water, eating factory-farmed poultry, and snacking on raisins to your little heart's content (*blackie!*)—then by now your body itself is a significant source of fluoride. As we have learned, fluoride accumulates in human bone, teeth, and other tissues. It is unknown how long fluoride remains in the body, but the National Research Council (NRC) of the National Academy of Sciences references a half-life of twenty years for fluoride contained in human bone.[1] That means it takes *twenty years* for just *half* of the fluoride you absorb into your bones today to be removed from your body.

The NRC admits this estimate might not reflect the true half-life of fluoride. There are so many variables involved that researchers are unable to determine the standard timeframe it takes for fluoride to be eliminated from human tissue. Admittedly, they have not tried very hard. The CDC does not include fluoride in its national biomonitoring surveys or nutritional studies.

But we don't need to know the average half-life of fluoride. I can think of many questions that are more helpful than trying to ascertain a national average. For example, what is the mechanism that causes the human body to eliminate fluoride? What other factors are involved? Is there a way to accelerate the process? Does fluoride cause the same symptoms on the way out as it does on the way in? If so, how can those symptoms be ameliorated?

There is a paucity of information on how to detoxify fluoride, but my obsessive intelligence analyst brain would not let me rest until I figured it out. Piecing together information gleaned from online forums, Internet, and small pockets of researchers in India, China, Africa, Canada and here in the United States, a general framework for how to detoxify fluoride from living tissue starts to become apparent.

The most important data, of course, is how this information influences bodies in the physical world. I will tell you my experience with fluoride detoxification, but because this topic is so poorly studied, you will have to make some important decisions on how *and if* you will venture down this path.

It is possible to heal acne completely simply by avoiding certain foods and beverages. If that is your health goal, there is no need to proceed further. Case solved. But for me, after I realized my acne (and depression) was caused by fluoride, I started wondering if it was possible to eliminate enough fluoride from my body so I would no

---

[1] *"Fluoride in Drinking Water: A Scientific Review of EPA's Standards,"* National Research Council of the National Academies, 2006, p. 92.

longer be sensitive to it. If I reduced the amount of fluoride in my body, would I be acne-proof? I also started wondering what other health effects I might experience in the future from fluoride that had already bioaccumulated in my bones, teeth, pineal gland, and who knows where else. Am I at a higher risk for arthritis? Cancer? What about my unborn children? Would it affect them? These questions were too important to let them linger. It was not easy, but I had to find answers. And find answers, I did.

*****

The Magic Dragon Who Lives By The Sea

My first lead came from a mysterious commenter called earthview who left a tip on my blog soon after I started writing about fluoride-induced acne. Earthview recommended I investigate the work of a small group of physicians who were collaborating on an initiative they referred to as "The Iodine Project." As earthview explained,

> *Since we get so little Iodine in our diets these days (unless you're into seaweed) we can start getting toxic build-ups of both fluoride and bromide in our systems — and both of these are toxic to our bodies. Dr. Guy Abraham has found that by increasing one's Iodine intake, the body starts to flush out the bromide and fluoride, and the Iodine takes up its proper place in its receptors. There are studies by Dr. Guy Abraham posted on the web, which include graphs of the results.*

I found one of the graphs in the studies earthview mentioned. It is a simple chart that shows urinary fluoride levels for each of six patients before, during, and after thirty days of supplementation with 37.5 mg of iodine per day.[2] The fluoride levels were lowest prior to taking the

---

[2] Abraham, G.E. "The historical background of the iodine project," *The Original Internist*, vol. 12, issue 2, 2005, pp.57-66.

supplement. On day one, they jumped to their highest point. On day 30, they were lower than on day one, but still significantly higher than before the iodine supplement was taken. This general trend across all six subjects seemed to support Abraham's assertion that the iodine supplement was displacing fluoride. I was intrigued enough to investigate further.

Before vanishing into the digital ether, earthview also mentions that iodine is used to treat fibrocystic disease of the ovaries and breast, and that perhaps it affects cystic disorders of the skin in a similar fashion. Like the reproductive organs, skin requires a significant amount of iodine for optimal health.

In his lecture at the annual Restorative Medicine Conference in 2011, Jorge Flechas, a practicing family physician in North Carolina and one of the two doctors involved in the initial Iodine Project, explains that conventional medical opinion is fixated on the use of iodine by the thyroid gland and neglects its critical role elsewhere in the body.[3] He and the other "Iodine Doctors," as they have come to be known, noticed that when their patients' body tissues lack iodine, the result is cysts, nodules, scar tissue, and pain. It happens in the breasts. It happens in the muscles. And although Flechas doesn't mention acne, he does mention that twenty percent of the total iodine content of the body is contained in the skin.

Cysts, nodules, scar tissue, and pain. Does that sound familiar? When Flechas works with his patients to correct their iodine deficiencies through supplementation, these symptoms are resolved.

I see we have a few dermatologists in the crowd who are dying to employ an old doctor's tactic (you probably saw this one before) where they butt in on our conversation by tossing out some studies from *the literature*[4] that supposedly disprove our burgeoning laymen theory that iodine is the ultimate antidote for fluoride. Even though

---

[3] View the lecture at ProjectFree.Me/Flechas.

[4] I feel like this term needs to be italicized to reflect the snooty accent with which I am using to say it. I'll stop.

dermatologists think diet does not cause acne, they almost unanimously agree that iodine *does* cause acne. They weasel around the diet connection because they only notice the phenomenon with iodine-based drugs and high amounts of seaweed that normal people don't eat (except for millions of people in other cultures who don't count for obvious reasons).[5]

As early as the 1960s, dermatologists noticed this connection between iodine and acne.[6] They are still super confused about how it works though, so we are going to have to explain it to them. To be nice, we should also give them a few tips for how they could have figured it out on their own by using some simple analytic techniques that seasoned analysts use to conduct analysis.

So, dermatologists are in widespread agreement that iodine can cause acne. That's great! Good job, guys. Now let's see if we can find any disconfirming evidence to help them grow their assessment. As I mentioned in the introduction, the CIA textbook on *Psychology of Intelligence Analysis* by Dick Heuer is required reading for intelligence analysts during basic training.[7] It should be required reading for medical researchers, too. From chapter four, Strategies for Analytical Judgment: "An optimal analytical strategy requires that analysts search for information to *disconfirm* their favorite theories, not employ a satisficing strategy that permits acceptance of the first hypothesis that seems consistent with the evidence" (emphasis added).

In intelligence analysis, analysts are instructed to intentionally look for disconfirming evidence and then not pooh-pooh it.[8] Managers

---

[5] I don't know why.

[6] Hitch, J.M.; Greenburg, B.G. "Adolescent Acne and Dietary Iodine," *Archives of Dermatology*, vol. 84, issue 6, 1961, pp. 898-911.

[7] You can read it for free at www.cia.gov/library/center-for-the-study-of-intelligence/csi-publications/books-and-monographs/psychology-of-intelligence-analysis/PsychofIntelNew.pdf.

[8] I forget the technical definition the Intelligence Community provides for pooh-poohing but you know what I mean. I hope this isn't foreshadowing that there are going to be fart jokes in this section. If so, I'm sorry in advance.

are advised to encourage dissenting viewpoints through devil's advocate exercises, interdisciplinary brainstorming, competitive analysis, intra-office peer review, and elicitation of outside expertise. They don't always do this (you know what they say—bureaucrats will be bureaucrats) but at least they are told that they should. I don't see that happening in government-sanctioned medicine where the stakes are magnified by the millions. This uncomfortable space of cognitive dissonance is where the analytic magic happens. It's what pushes us forward, forcing us to confront our misperceptions, refine our theories, and *learn* about the world.

Looking through the literature, it appears there are only a few researchers who put up any kind of fuss about iodine causing acne. In 1961, about ten years after most cities in North Carolina started fluoridating their water supply, two researchers from the University of North Carolina conducted a study to compare the rates of acne between adolescents who eat a lot of seafood on the coast, and those in the mountainous western region of the state where a diet rich in seafood and therefore iodine is less common.[9] The results of their study were not what anyone expected. The adolescents who consumed more iodine had *less* acne.

The researchers concluded that iodine does not cause acne, but everyone else pretty much ignored them because iodine-induced acne was already confirmed, and who cares about dietary causes of acne anyway. If the researchers allowed for a period of cognitive dissonance rather than drawing the hasty conclusion that iodine does not cause acne, they might have focused follow-up studies on trying to figure out why iodine seems to cause acne in some people but inhibit acne in others.

This observation is easily explained within the fluoride theory of acne. As Guy Abraham's studies show, the ingestion of dietary iodine causes fluoride to be released in urine. If iodine turns out to be

---

[9] Hitch, J.M.; Greenburg, B.G. "Adolescent Acne and Dietary Iodine," *Archives of Dermatology*, vol. 84, issue 6, 1961, pp. 898-911.

the antidote for fluoride, as I am proposing here, then consuming iodine on a regular basis would help limit the amount of fluoride that accumulates in your body, making you less susceptible to acne. However, if your body already contains significant amounts of fluoride and then you consume a large dose of iodine, the amount of fluoride released back into your circulation can cause acne just as it does when you consume too much fluoride in a glass of water.

My anecdotal experience with iodine supports this theory. I developed breakouts from seaweed, fish eggs, and iodine supplements.[10] I never had a reaction from fish or shellfish which contain significantly less iodine than seaweed.

Another piece of disconfirming evidence that iodine causes acne was uncovered in 2006, when William Danby from Dartmouth Medical School pointed out that iodine might not cause "true acne" because "the hallmark of acne, the comedo, is not part of the initial lesion."[11] *Comedo* is the Latin term formerly used for flesh-eating worms, but dermatologists stole it to use as their secret codename for blocked pores since blackheads remind them of little black worms secreting from your skin.

The initial acne caused by iodine doesn't have a blocked pore. Just pus.[12] This observation disconfirms the widely-held theory that acne is caused by clogged pores but it makes perfect sense in our theory that acne is caused by fluoride. If dermatologists had pursued this piece of evidence they might have been forced to admit that clogged pores are correlated with acne, but they do not cause it.

(While Danby suggests the comedo is the hallmark of true acne, I would like to propose that the hallmark of true acne is zits. The

---

[10] Perhaps the reaction I had to anchovies was because they contained iodine, not fluoride. I am still not clear on this one. Usually the iodine-induced breakouts take longer to show up, though.

[11] Danby, William F. "Acne and iodine: Reply," *Journal of the American Academy of Dermatology,* vol. 56, issue 1, Jan 2007, pp. 164-165.

[12] Jackson, Robert. "Non-bacterial pus-forming diseases of the skin," *Canadian Medical Association Journal,* vol. 111, issue 8, Oct 19, 1974, pp. 801, 804-806.

term "zit" first appeared in dictionaries in 1966 following the widespread fluoridation of the public water supply. The etymology is unknown. Zit only means one thing, and every American knows what it is.)

So how much iodine does it take to displace toxic fluoride from your body? Oh boy, does that question open a can of comedones! The government's Recommended Daily Allowance of iodine is 150 to 290 micrograms per day. The Iodine Doctors argue the optimal dose is roughly *one hundred times* that amount, and often higher if your body is storing toxic halides such as bromide and fluoride.

Of all the competing arguments in modern medicine, this is one of the most controversial ideas I've encountered. Mainstream physicians will tell you this amount of iodine can kill you, or at least permanently damage vulnerable thyroid tissue. Even some of my favorite "alternative" health docs such as Joe Mercola and Chris Kresser are wary of recommending this amount of iodine in the absence of further studies. Paleo dieters conclude this amount of iodine wasn't a traditional part of the paleolithic diet and is therefore undesirable.[13]

Real world experiences of people supplementing with iodine don't help to clarify the matter. When Sally Fallon of the Weston Price Foundation and Katie from Wellness Mama tried iodine supplementation, they both experienced negative reactions and decided iodine was not right for them.

And yet, the Iodine Doctors point out that iodine supplements were widely consumed in these amounts since the discovery of iodine two hundred years ago. Moreover, they successfully treat thousands of patients in their clinics through iodine supplementation each year and are easily able to measure fluoride and bromide released in urine after iodine is ingested. Thriving communities of iodine discussion forums

---

[13] In intelligence analysis, we call this logic "mirror-imaging," where your assessment of how other cultures think and behave is unduly influenced by underlying assumptions of how people in your own culture think and behave. More on this later.

on Yahoo and Curezone support their claims as people share their experiences of how iodine healed various health crises.

How do we reconcile these viewpoints that seem to exist in direct conflict with each other? From chapter eight of *Psychology of Intelligence Analysis*: "Analysis of competing hypotheses (ACH) requires an analyst to explicitly identify all the reasonable alternatives and have them compete against each other for the analyst's favor, rather than evaluating their plausibility one at a time." Brainstorming a variety of alternative hypotheses for a certain scenario is a handy way to become aware of possibilities you might not otherwise consider. Let's try it.

What are some of the possible hypotheses with iodine supplementation? It is possible the official view of iodine is correct and amounts over 1 mg are potentially dangerous. Another hypothesis is that the Iodine Doctors are correct, and the body requires 13+ mg for optimal health. A third option is that neither of them are correct. Maybe amounts over 1 mg aren't dangerous, but the human body does not need that much iodine anyway. A fourth option is that they are both correct: amounts of iodine over 1 milligram are potentially dangerous, but the body requires 13+ milligrams for optimal health. Are you feeling some cognitive dissonance with that last one? That's a good sign.[14]

Keeping these competing hypotheses in mind, we can now move on to the evidence. And not just the scientific evidence. Restricting our assessment to the scientific evidence would severely limit our analysis. From fluoridation to acne to raisins to mink oil, the controversies we covered in this book provide a game plan for how to approach this type of hazy health information. First we look at tradition and the historical precedent. How were people using iodine prior to the modern era when bureaucrats and billion dollar industries gained a virtual monopoly on scientific consensus? Next, how did the

---

[14] There are a lot more possible hypotheses here; I'm just trying to keep things simple for the M.D.s ;)

tradition change? Who were the players involved and what were the stakes? By studying the story of iodine, we understand the science in a new light.

Iodine was discovered in 1811 when a Frenchman was creating potassium nitrate to make gunpowder during the Napoleonic wars. The customary French method for making potassium nitrate was to use wood ash mixed with feces and urine to let it decompose for a year. Excrement was abundant in Napoleonic France but after several years of war, wood ash was scarce so French manufacturers started burning seaweed instead.

One such Frenchman, a prior pharmacist and chemist named Bernard Courtois, was investigating corrosion on his copper vessels when he noticed that sulfuric acid added to seaweed ash gave off a plume of violet vapor that condensed as solid crystals the color and luster of graphite. When substances transition directly between gas and solid forms like this, without an intermediate liquid state, it is known as a process called sublimation. Corroded copper vessels, a flash of a violet vapor, sublimation, lustrous crystals—how is chemistry *not* magic? The mysterious element was given the name iodine from the Greek word *ioeides*, meaning violet-colored.

Soon after he discovered iodine, Courtois began discussing the element with his pharmacist friends and provided samples for them to study. In less than a decade, physicians throughout Europe were using iodine to treat a common condition called goiter, an enlargement of the thyroid gland that was previously treated with burnt sea sponges. Iodine quickly earned a reputation for healing a variety of other ailments, from asthma and ulcers to joint disease and deafness. It proved to have seemingly miraculous antiseptic properties, too. Gauze strips saturated in iodine were hung from the crossbeams in European hospitals. Seaweed was strewn across the floor. People wore small vials of iodine around their neck and Civil War soldiers carried iodine canteens as an essential part of their gear. In a letter to his brother,

Vincent Van Gogh raved about iodine as a treatment for syphilis.[15]

By the twentieth century, iodine was widely known as a panacea. Albert Szent-Gyorgyi, the Nobel prize-winning physiologist who discovered vitamin C in the 1930s, described iodine as "the universal medicine." In his biography, he even quotes a little rhyme that was commonly repeated about potassium iodide in medical school, "If you don't know what, where or why, prescribe ye then K and I." Potassium iodide is the most popular form of iodine, especially a liquid solution called Lugol's that is still available today.

By the 1920s, scientists were in agreement that not only does iodine heal goiter, but it also prevents it. It seems obvious now, but the idea that iodine deficiency leads to goiter was suggested throughout the previous century and repeatedly rejected because measuring methods for determining the iodine content of food, soil, and other relevant substances were new and untrusted, making it difficult to prove that iodine deficiency was the culprit. Many researchers at the time favored the idea of a "toxic agent" to explain the cause of goiter. What no one seemed to realize is that these two theories are not mutually exclusive.

In 1924, the United States began a salt iodization program in Michigan, the future birthplace of fluoridation and the heart of the American "goiter belt" which comprised the Great Lakes, Appalachia, and the northwest. During World War I, Michigan doctors demonstrated that in some parts of the state, as many as 60 percent of men eligible for the draft had enlarged necks due to goiter, many of whom were disqualified from the military as a result.[16] After iodide was added to salt, the incidence of goiter plummeted.

Iodine's popularity in the first half of the twentieth century is hard to imagine today. South Carolina license plates proudly displayed

---

[15] For more info on the history of iodine, see Lynne Farrow's book, *The Iodine Crisis: What You Don't Know About Iodine Can Wreck Your Life*, Devon Press, 2013.

[16] Leung, A.M.; Braverman, L.E.; Pearce, E.N., "History of U.S. Iodine Fortification and Supplementation," *Nutrients*, vol 4, issue 11, 2012, pp. 1740–1746.

the phrase "The Iodine State" because of the high iodine content of the soil there. Championship swimmers preferred pools treated with iodine over those with chlorine.[17] By mid century, iodine was added to baked goods as a dough conditioner. A single slice of bread contained the full Recommended Daily Allowance of 150 micrograms of iodine. Combined with iodine from eggs, milk, vegetables, seafood, and iodized salt, it becomes clear that many Americans were consuming much more than the recommended amount. Doctors treating patients with asthma described 300 *milligrams* of iodine as a "low" dose,[18] and often used doses in the gram amounts on large numbers of patients for several years at a time with good results.[19]

Within a few decades, iodine was quietly removed from baked goods. We have since forgotten it can be used to treat swimming pools. Few people store a bottle of it in their bathroom cabinet these days, let alone around their neck. And when doctors don't know what, where or why, no one ever told them to prescribe K and I.

This brings us to our next question. In the latter half of the twentieth century, why did a genuine essential nutrient that was so highly regarded since its discovery suddenly vanish from our doctors' medicine bags? What changed the historical precedent? To be honest, this part is boring. I'm tired of writing about bureaucrats and their institutionally entrenched viewpoints, and I am already *freaking out* over our grand finale in the next sections. As much as I want to skip ahead, this part of the story is vital. We need to know where we came from to understand where we are. And we need to understand where we are before we can figure out how to get where we want to go.

---

[17] Abraham, G.E., "The safe and effective implementation of orthoiodosupplementation in medical practice," *The Original Internist*, issue 11, 2004, pp. 17-36.

[18] Bernecker, C. "Intermittent therapy with potassium iodide in chronic obstructive disease of the airways," A*cta Allergologica*, vol. 24, 1969, pp. 216-225.

[19] Abraham, G.E., "The safe and effective implementation of orthoiodosupplementation in medical practice," *The Original Internist*, issue 11, 2004, pp. 17-36.

Okay, where were we. I have a feeling we were about to discuss another old white guy? Oh right, Theodore Kocher. He was a physician and professor for 45 years at the University of Bern, one of the five university hospitals in Switzerland. Kocher somehow dodged all the malpractice lawsuits he likely encountered while experimenting with thyroidectomies in the late nineteenth century and instead won the Nobel Prize in 1909 for his surgical techniques that reduced the mortality rate of thyroid surgery. (Just spitballing here, but perhaps he was able to maintain his reputation by taking credit for the discovery that the full thyroidectomies he pioneered result in cretinism. Kocher published an article on the topic in 1883 while failing to acknowledge the Swiss researchers who published a paper on the same condition the year prior and first reported it to him in 1972.)[20]

Kocher was the first surgeon to ever win the Nobel Prize and was considered a leading figure in the field of surgery at the time. He was also an outspoken critic of the use of iodine to treat patients with hyperthyroidism. Not surprisingly, he endorsed the technique he developed for thyroid surgery instead. Because of his influence in the medical community, many thyroidologists stopped using iodine for goiters associated with hyperthyroidism and it ceased to even be a topic of discussion within the Royal Society of Medicine.

After Kocher's death in 1917, physicians at Mayo Clinic and elsewhere started reporting high success rates using Lugol's solution for hyperthyroid patients and thus its reputation was reinstated.[21] Iodine narrowly escaped vivisection from the Swiss master surgeon, but the field we would soon come to know as "modern medicine" had another hitman waiting in the laboratory wings.

Jan Wolff was a young undergraduate student when he joined Israel Chaikoff's laboratory at University of California at Berkeley in

---

[20] https://en.wikipedia.org/wiki/Emil_Theodor_Kocher

[21] Abraham, G.E., "The safe and effective implementation of orthoiodosupplementation in medical practice," *The Original Internist*, issue 11, 2004, pp. 17-36.

the mid-1940s. In 1948, with Chaikoff as a co-author, Wolff published a short paper entitled, "The Inhibitory Action of Iodide on Organic Binding of Iodine by the Normal Thyroid Gland."[22] The whole article was less than two pages long but its main assertion is still screwing with women's hormones today.

In the study, Wolff injected rats with varying dosages of potassium iodide labeled with a radioisotope of iodine discovered at Berkeley a few years prior. Over the next 50 hours, he observed how the iodine was absorbed by the rats' thyroid glands by removing them at designated intervals, grinding them up in miniature rat thyroid blenders, and then measuring their iodine content with a Geiger-Muller counter. Wolff concluded, "[T]hyroid tissue is inhibited by iodine regardless of its state of activity." Unlike Kocher, Wolff wasn't just referring to cases of overactive thyroid glands. He was referring to thyroid glands in general.

Another principle from Dick Heuer's *Psychology of Intelligence Analysis* is called for here. Like a well-crafted haiku, its words are simple but compelling. From chapter six, Keeping an Open Mind: "The principle of deferred judgment is undoubtedly the most important."

If a Berkeley grad student wants to inject perfectly congenial rodents with radioactive iodine and then put their thyroids in a Vitamix to measure the iodine content, fine. (It's not actually fine, but we really don't have time to get into that here.)[23] But would it not be prudent to defer judgment on the dramatic conclusion that iodine, an essential nutrient, inhibits healthy thyroid function until more information can be gathered? Such as, what happens with continued iodine exposure after 50 hours? Do injections with radioactive iodine produce a different affect than forms of dietary iodine? Is decreased

---

[22] Wolff, J.; Chaikoff, I.L. "The inhibitory action of iodide upon organic binding of iodine by the normal thyroid gland," *The Journal of Biological Chemistry*, vol. 172, issue 2, 1948, pp.855-856.

[23] See www.washingtonpost.com/national/health-science/a-new-model-of-empathy-the-rat/2011/12/08/gIQAAx0jfO_story.html.

absorption of radioactive iodine a bad thing? Do these fluctuations in thyroid hormone make the rat feel *bad*? Oh, and how does this information translate to other species, say, hominids for example?

No, Wolff doesn't identify any of these intelligence gaps in his article. Instead, he declares, and I repeat, "Thus thyroid tissue is inhibited by iodine regardless of its state of activity." The young Wolff draws that judgment right there in his very first paper on iodine supplementation. Such a dramatic statement turned out to be a great career move, but what about the rest of humanity?

Wolff continued to study the thyroid gland throughout his long and illustrious career in endocrinology, but as the bottom line of his 1948 paper revealed, he already made a hasty judgment. Once that mental model is in place, it is difficult to see the world any other way. As Heuer explains, "[W]hether it manifests itself as self-censorship of one's own ideas or fear of critical evaluation by colleagues or supervisors... New ideas are, by definition, unconventional, and therefore likely to be suppressed, either consciously or unconsciously."

Here is where Wolff and the endocrinology community in general make another big analytic error. Instead of looking for disconfirming evidence to grow their understanding of how iodine affects the thyroid gland, they then focused on evidence that confirmed the hasty judgment that was already made. They noticed that in communities where salt iodization programs were established to prevent severe iodine deficiency, there was a rise in a certain form of hyperthyroidism.[24] That evidence fits nicely into their theory, so they used it to justify their preexisting belief that iodine inhibits thyroid function.

They also noticed that the rate of hyperthyroidism sometimes dropped below previous levels after a few years of salt iodization, as was the case in Switzerland in the 1980s, and that increases in dietary iodine other than from iodized salt sometimes do not result in more

---

[24] Stanbury, J.B. et al. "Iodine-Induced Hyperthyroidism: Occurrence and Epidemiology," *Thyroid*, vol. 8, issue 1, 1998.

reports of hyperthyroidism, as was the case in the United States in the 1960s.[25] This evidence does not fit with their theory, so most endocrinologists mention it only in passing if at all, missing out on a valuable opportunity to refine their current understanding of the world.

If endocrinologists had allowed disconfirming evidence about iodine into their analysis, they might have eventually realized that other variables influence how iodine affects the thyroid gland, such as the presence of nutritional cofactors and goitrogens like fluoride. Instead they cling to an over-simplistic theory developed by the big bureaucrat on campus while he was still in graduate school.

Wolff's theory that iodine inhibits healthy thyroid function came to be known as the Wolff-Chaikoff effect and is still seen as a major regulator of thyroid function. In 1969, Wolff published a review of all the evidence that confirms his theory on the pharmacologic effects of excess iodine. He proposed that the estimated daily iodine requirement "for man" (*eye roll*) is only 200 mcg since that is the amount he suggests is required by the thyroid gland.[26]

The Wolff-Chaikoff effect is the reason iodine was removed from baked goods.[27] It is the reason the American Thyroid Association warns against iodine consumption greater than 1 milligram,[28] a small fraction of what many societies healthier than ours consume on a daily basis. It is also the reason the Recommended Daily Allowance for

---

[25] *Ibid.*

[26] "Since the normal human thyroid gland delivers about 65 mcg of organic iodine (T3 and T4) to the circulation per day, and since the iodide clearance of the thyroid is half that of the kidneys, a rough estimate of the daily iodide requirement for man would be about 200 mcg of iodine per day. Approximately 10 per cent of this is derived from deiodination of secreted organic iodine and the remainder from the diet." Source: Wolff, Jan. "Iodide goiter and the pharmacologic effects of excess iodide," *The American Journal of Medicine,* vol. 47, issue 1, Jul 1969, pp. 101–124.

[27] And also, because thyroid glands that contain iodine make it difficult for doctors to read radioactive iodine scans. See http://iodinehistory.blogspot.com/2015/02/i-was-right.html.

[28] www.thyroid.org/ata-statement-on-the-potential-risks-of-excess-iodine-ingestion-and-exposure/

iodine was set at 150 micrograms instead of at the level the human body needs to avoid iodine deficiencies other than simple goiter.

Since Wolff is an endocrinologist focused on the thyroid gland, he does not consider the iodine requirements of other organs. But how much iodine is needed by the ovaries, mammary glands, muscles, skin, and other essential body parts? The National Institute of Health's Endocrine Biochemistry Section, which Wolff directed as recently as 2008, has no idea because they never conducted those studies.

Wolff's half-century tenure as a government bureaucrat at NIH is an important part of our story. The National Institute of Health is the largest biomedical research agency in the world. It spends over 30 billion American dollars on medical research each year, most of which is awarded to universities, medical schools, and other research institutions around the globe. As you now know, Wolff—one of the founding members of the endocrinology branch at NIH who worked his way to chief of the Endocrine Biochemistry Section—established his very name and reputation on the Wolff-Chaikoff effect, which was used to denigrate iodine.

If you were an endocrinologist seeking funding for your research, would you choose to investigate the validity of the Wolff-Chaikoff effect by studying the benefits of an inexpensive, non-patentable nutritional supplement? How would that conversation go? "Hi there, Mr. Wolff. Can I have some money to show that your whole career is based on a fallacy and you've unwittingly caused suffering and death for millions of people? Please let me know what you think. Tha-anks!"

I'm sure Mr. Wolff is a very nice person and my intention is not to malign his name. But these are human lives we are talking about, not beakers and test tubes. *Clap, clap!* Get your head in the game, *Jan!*

There's another reason the Wolff-Chaikoff effect is still standing and it's soooo cliché I don't even feel like talking about it. You probably already know the gist of this story, but we still need to go there so... Guess who was behind the denigration of dietary iodine.

Dentists?? Good guess, but no. It was another one of our story's big villains. The reason the Wolff-Chaikoff effect gained traction like it did was because of the drug lords, of course, and I'm not referring to dermatologists this time.

When Wolff started studying iodine in the mid-1940s, researchers were investigating a relatively new approach to treating hyperthyroidism. Instead of nourishing an unhealthy thyroid gland with seaweed or iodine as was the practice since the dawn of recorded history (and probably prior), doctors began attacking overactive thyroid glands with goiter-causing substances, known as goitrogens, in an effort to force them to stop overacting and behave as good little thyroids should.

Two such "anti-thyroid" medications, thiourea and thiouracil, were introduced in 1943 by a Harvard researcher named E.B. Astwood. These goitrogens would later evolve into the family of thionamides that doctors employ to assail thyroid glands today, such as methimazole (brand name Tapazole) and propylthiouracil. Wolff's paper was published five years after Astwood introduced these antithyroid medications to the world.

Wolff's study involved rats, as we know, but less than one year later Malcolm Stanley from Tufts University published a study extending the Wolff-Chaikoff effect to humans.[29] This study was the evidence NIH pointed to in the 1960s when they figured out bakeries were using iodine as a dough conditioner and first expressed concern that it was significantly adding to the total dietary intake of iodine for most Americans.[30] By the 1970s, bread manufacturers began using bromide in place of iodine.

As you might recall from our periodic chart, bromide is a halogen that sits above iodine on the table of the elements. Like

---

[29] Stanley, M.M. "The direct estimation of the rate of thyroid hormone formation in man. The effect of the iodide ion on thyroid iodine utilization." *Journal of Clinical Endocrinology*, vol. 9, 1949, pp. 941-954.

[30] London, W.T.; Vought, R.L.; Brown, F.A. "Bread—a dietary source of large quantities of iodine," *New England Journal of Medicine*, vol. 273, issue 7, 1965.

fluoride, it is a known goitrogen that depresses thyroid function. Brominated flour has since been banned in Europe, Canada, Brazil, Argentina, Peru, China, South Korea, Sri Lanka, Nigeria and probably a bunch of other countries because *it causes thyroid cancer*.[31] In the United States, however, the FDA only "discourages"[32] manufacturers from using brominated flour which of course does not prevent it from showing up in your Tastykakes.

It is unclear how Mr. Stanley was able to conduct human trials on the Wolff-Chaikoff effect, analyze the data, write a paper, submit it for publication, and have it published in a major medical journal only one year after Wolff's study was published. It is likely he had inside information about Wolff's line of research. There is nothing wrong with that, but it suggests there was some kind of relationship between the two researchers or that they worked together in some way. And who else did Stanley work with? E.B. Astwood, the man who introduced anti-thyroid pharmaceuticals just a few years prior.

Astwood and Stanley both worked at Tufts University at the time Stanley's paper extending the Wolff-Chaikoff effect to humans was published. Astwood is not listed as a coauthor on Stanley's paper, but in the requisite memoir written to enshrine his name in the community of science saints, Astwood's colleagues explain, "Because of his modesty, Astwood's name was withheld from many of the pioneering publications on the thyroid that came from his laboratory, even though he supplied the funds and space and contributed to the development of the ideas that generated the studies. Such self-effacement is uncommon among scientists."[33] Astwood and Stanley authored another paper together that same year about using

---

[31] DeAngelo, A.B. et al. "Carcinogenicity of potassium bromate administered in the drinking water to male B6C3F1 mice and F344/N rats," *Journal of Toxicologic Pathology*, vol. 26, issue 5, 1998, pp. 587-594.

[32] www.newsweek.com/five-controversial-food-additives-83551

[33] Greep, Roy O.; Greer, Monty A. "Edwin Bennett Astwood, 1909—1976: A Biographical Memoir," *National Academy of Sciences*, 1985.

goitrogenic drugs as an alternative treatment to iodine for
hyperthyroidism.[34]

Once the anti-thyroid drug manufacturers established their
footing in the pharmaceutical world, there was no turning back from
the Wolff-Chaikoff myth. As we've seen before, the industries that
grow up around a government institutionalized blunder serve as
patrons for its propagation and sustainment. Like fluoridation and
fluoristan toothpaste. Or vintage federal legislation and the beauty
industry. Or the Raisin Reserve and puppy murderers.

Thyroid medication is serious business. The hypothyroid drug
levothyroxine, also known as Synthroid, is consistently listed as the
most frequently prescribed pharmaceutical in the United States.[35] If a
scientific consensus developed around the idea that thyroid disorders
are best treated through increased consumption of iodine and
decreased exposure to goitrogens, the industry would crumble. How
could humble little iodine be expected to clear its name in the face of
such a giant adversary?

Despite the government egos and industry interests vested in
thyroid research, the occasional pro-iodine study still makes its way
into the published literature like an SBDF in church.[36] When it
happens, most people just try to ignore it and keep looking straight
ahead. But on occasion, someone turns around and says, "What
stinks?"

In 1993, Bill Ghent published a study in which 1,365 women
with fibrocystic breast disease consumed 5 milligrams of dietary
iodine per day for approximately one year.[37] The results showed a

----

[34] Stanley, M.M.; Astwood, E.B. "1-Methyl-2-mercaptoimidazole; an antithyroid
compound highly active in man," *Endocrinology*, vol. 44, issue 6, 1949, p. 588.

[35] Brown, Troy. "The 10 Most-Prescribed and Top-Selling Medications," *Medscape
Medical News*, May 8, 2015.

[36] And there it is.

[37] Ghent, W.R. et. al. "Iodine Replacement in Fibrocystic Disease of the Breast,"
Canadian Journal of Surgery, vol. 36, 1993, pp. 453-460.

significant reduction in fibrosis and no indication of the much-hyped Wolff-Chaikoff effect, even though Wolff predicted that daily amounts of iodine of 2 milligrams were "excessive and potentially harmful."[38]

Like Wolff, Ghent was a bit of a big wig himself—but in Canada where he served as Chairman of the Canadian Medical Association's Health Care Council. His article appeared in the *Canadian Journal of Surgery*, which helps explain why he was one of the few researchers to share the results of a study aboot "high dose" iodine supplementation, eh? Unfortunately for iodine, Ghent died three months before the study was published, leaving him little opportunity to promote his findings or conduct further investigation.

Ghent might have dealt it, but Abraham smelt it.[39] Guy Abraham was a retired professor of obstetrics, gynecology and endocrinology at the UCLA School of Medicine. In the 1970s, he pioneered the development of methods to measure minute quantities of steroid hormones in biological fluids. In the 1980s, after realizing that premenstrual tension was an early indicator of more serious gynecologic disorders, he developed nutritional programs to alleviate PMS (so yes, Guy Abraham is a bona fide science saint).

Retired and living the good life in California in the 1990s, Abraham happened to read Ghent's paper on iodine supplementation a few years after it was published. He found it odd that Ghent reported such positive results with doses of iodine that were over twice as high as what American doctors were told was the safe limit. Abraham started researching the literature on iodine supplementation and found that studies were prolific prior to the 1940s, but mysteriously disappeared when goitrogenic drugs and a certain "famous thyroidologist" took the stage.

When Guy Abraham learned that 60 million people in Japan were eating iodine-rich seaweed every day without any indication of

---

[38] Wolff, J. "Iodide Goiter and the Parmacologic Effects of Excess Iodide," *American Journal of Medicine*, vol. 47, 1969, pp. 101-124.

[39] You're right. I need to stop the fart allusions. It's weird.

the Wolff-Chaikoff effect in action, he decided it was time to investigate the theory more directly. Using his own funding, he teamed with Jorge Flechas, the family physician in North Carolina mentioned earlier, to perform a few pilot studies and then a larger study of ten women to see if the results would confirm Ghent's observations.[40] They did, so he funded longer and larger studies, adding Michigan-based family physician David Brownstein to his team in the process. The Iodine Doctors did not see any signs of the Wolff-Chaikoff effect in their patients. Instead, all the evidence supported the hypothesis that the human body requires milligrams of iodine on a daily basis, not micrograms.[41]

I never met Guy Abraham to confirm this, but at this point of the story you can sense his blood pressure rising. He spent his whole career at UCLA studying women's health issues like fibromyalgia and ovarian tumors. After realizing the entire population of women he was treating was iodine deficient for the sad reasons described in this chapter, and that simply correcting their iodine deficiency could lead to the resolution of many of the conditions he studied, Abraham felt **"grossly deceived"** by the national medical establishment he had been a part of for 35 years. (That's his bold print there, not mine.)

Guy Abraham was mad. And what happens when old, retired people get mad? Because I live in Florida, I know this one: they rant. It's *awesome*. Abraham published many articles in stodgy peer-reviewed journals throughout his career—*Obstetrics & Gynecology, The Journal of Reproductive Medicine, The Journal of Clinical Endocrinology & Metabolism, The American Journal of Clinical Nutrition*, etc. But in retirement, without an institution like UCLA attached to his name, he was able to spread his literary wings to really speak his mind.

Abraham started publishing research from his Iodine Project in

[40] Abraham, G.E.; Flechas, J.D.; Hakala, J.C., "Optimum Levels of Iodine for Greatest Mental and Physical Health," *The Original Internist*, vol. 9, 2002, pp. 5-20.

[41] To see their full collection of published studies from 2002 to 2008, visit www.optimox.com/iodine-research.

a small natural health care journal called *The Original Internist*. As with the articles he wrote earlier in his career, they are still heavy on the science, but there's a distinct retiree tone that only people of a certain age can pull off.

To give a few examples, Abraham documents a new condition called medical iodophobia when medicoiodophobes suffer from double standards, doublethink, doublespeak, and contradictory logic.[42] He associates it with domestic bioterrorism and renames Wolff's theory "the Wolff-Chaikoff Iodophobic Domino Effect."[43] (I just noticed that abbreviates to Wolff-CIDE. Haha! Good one, Abraham.) Each of his articles has as many as five exclamation points, sometimes two in a row. Furthermore, on occasion, he *might* use the word "zombifying" in place of "goitrogenic" and there are a few teeeeensy references to Lucifer, the flood, Adam and Eve, Old Testament Bible verses, and a link at the bottom of each article for a "Praise the Lord" 14" x 18" poster free of charge. So what? The man was clearly onto something.

But then in February 2013, Guy Abraham fell, hit his head, and made his quiet departure from the world. He didn't leave much information about himself behind. There are no "about me" pages or saccharine memorials written by his medical disciples. Judging from the lone black and white photograph posted of him online, that was probably the way he wanted it.

In generations past, Abraham's death might have spelled the end of his Iodine Project. But generations past didn't have a sidekick named Internet. She was smart enough to hold on to his articles.[44] She also created a discursive space for people to share stories about his work. Then she sent earthview to whisper about it in my ear.

---

[42] Abraham, G.E., "The History of Iodine in Medicine Part III: Thyroid Fixation and Medical Iodophobia," *The Original Internist*, vol. 13, Jun 2006, pp. 71-78, June 2006.

[43] Abraham, G.E.,"The Wolff-Chaikoff Effect: Crying Wolf?" *The Original Internist*, vol. 12, issue 3, 2005, pp. 112-118.

[44] You can read them at www.optimox.com/iodine-research.

"Today, the public relies heavily on the Internet for health information... Control of health information on the Internet by iodophobic bioterrorists is a real threat to a population who depends on this source of information to make health-related decisions. Such a population is vulnerable and most likely will end up adopting iodophobic decisions to their detriment... Iodophobic bioterrorism can be prevented through education of health care professionals and the public at large. Remember that the easiest and most effective way to destroy a nation is the removal of iodine from the food supply. Iodophobic bioterrorism is a real threat to our nation, and the enemies within our gates masquerade as guardians of our thyroid gland."[45]

—Guy E. Abraham
? - 2013

*****

---

[45] Abraham, G.E.,"The Wolff-Chaikoff Effect: Crying Wolf?" *The Original Internist,* vol. 12, issue 3, 2005, pp. 112-118.

If I Only Had a Brain

The story of iodine described in the previous section is an edited version of its history. It can be no other way. But at least now you have an idea of how over the last two hundred years iodine was discovered, prized, vilified, forgotten and then discovered again. We learned it was widely used by doctors and individuals before government agencies endorsed pharmaceutical options in its place. Now we can move on to the most important question in our assessment of the conflicting health information surrounding iodine: what do our direct observations of the physical world tell us?

To answer this question for himself, Guy Abraham collaborated with two family physicians to incorporate iodine supplementation into their clinics. After learning that iodine displaced fluoride in their patients' lab tests, I decided it was time to answer the question for myself, too.

Like a kid trying to jump on a merry-go-round spinning just a little too fast, I fell on my face a few times when I first started supplementing with iodine. Because I don't want you to make the same mistakes I made, here are the biggest lessons I learned from all the dumb and counterproductive things I did *before* the time I finally jumped straight on.

*****

Lesson #1: Don't Start Here

Once you learn that iodine detoxifies fluoride, you might be tempted to rush out and buy some kombu or a bottle of kelp capsules and just see how things go. That's not a good idea. When I first learned that iodine displaces fluoride, I was still in the phase where I was figuring out exactly how to avoid fluoride in my diet. My skin was mostly acne-free because I had cut out the major offenders, but there were still some sneaky sources of fluoride making their way in. This was not the appropriate time to throw a couple of kelp tablets into the mix, but that is what I did. It took longer than I care to admit to realize the kelp pills were causing more acne. I was so focused on rooting out fluoride, I nearly missed it. They also caused persistent water retention, especially around my upper abdomen. If you are going to attempt to detoxify fluoride, *wait until you completely heal your acne* and you are confident you know how to limit your exposure to fluoride.

Lesson # 2: Food Isn't Always the Best Medicine

Since the kelp supplement didn't work out well for me, I returned to my old mantra of trying to obtain all the nutrients my body needs from food. I learned that fish eggs are nutrient-dense sources of iodine commonly eaten in traditional diets, so I started incorporating them into my breakfast each morning. Even the smallest of servings left me bloated and with breakouts. I tried seaweed snacks too, but had similar results. I eventually concluded that *food sources of iodine are not the best option for fluoride detoxification in fluoride-sensitive individuals* because it is nearly impossible to control the dose. As you'll see, controlling the amount of iodine you consume is critical.

Lesson # 3: Outsource

Next, I decided to try an actual iodine supplement. It was a very small dose, only slightly larger than the Recommended Daily Allowance. Again I developed acne and even more water retention which this time spread to my calves. A couple other unpleasant side effects were added to the list, too. For the first time in my life, I woke up with an excruciating cramp in my left foot. I also developed heart palpitations. Reminder: I am demonstrating what *not* to do at home.

Effective iodine supplementation is more complicated than simply popping iodine pills. This is why all the books and articles you will read about iodine supplementation recommend that you *work with an "iodine-literate" healthcare practitioner* to safely use iodine to detoxify fluoride.[46] While that advice sounds reasonable, the problem is that there are not many "iodine-literate" healthcare practitioners out there. I could not find one within several hours' drive even though I was living in a major metropolitan center at the time, so I gave up on iodine and started pursuing another lead on fluoride detoxification.

Lesson #4: The Prune Empire Strikes Back

Boron has also been found to detoxify fluoride, but I can't recommend it. The research is sparse, but in one study from 1987, Chinese researchers used borax to treat 31 patients suffering from skeletal fluorosis.[47] After administering increasing doses of borax, they measured the fluoride in the patients' urine against that of a control group and concluded that borax is an effective way to eliminate fluoride. Other studies on rats[48] and rabbits[49] draw the same conclusion. The online forum, EarthClinic, has a popular thread on using borax to detoxify fluoride, but I was skeptical of ingesting a substance I currently use to clean my toilet. Instead of borax, I tried a boron supplement. Even half the recommended dose resulted in acne and bloating, but then I also developed abdominal cramping, nausea, diarrhea, weakness, and dizziness—all signs of acute fluoride toxicity.

---

[46] Lynne Farrow, founder of Breast Cancer Choices, a non profit organization dedicated to educating women about the use of iodine therapy, maintains a list of iodine-literate physicians on her website at www.breastcancerchoices.org/ipractitioners.html.

[47] Zhou, L.Y. et al., "Effect of borax in treatment of skeletal fluorosis," *Fluoride*, vol 20, issue 1, 1987, pp. 24-27.

[48] Marcovitch, S.; Stanley, W.W. "A Study of Antidotes for Fluorine," *The Journal of Pharmacology and Experimental Therapeutic*, vol. 74, issue 2, 1942, pp. 235-8.

[49] Elsair, J. et al. "Boron as antidote to fluoride: effect on bones and claws in subacute intoxication of rabbits," *Fluoride*, vol. 14, issue 1, 1981, pp. 21-9.

Elsair, J. et al. "Boron as an antidote in acute fluoride intoxication in rabbits: its action on the fluoride and calcium-phosphorous metabolism," *Fluoride*, vol. 13, issue 1, 1980, pp. 30-38.

I was smart enough to stop taking boron, but dumb enough to try it again on two separate occasions to verify it was the boron that caused my symptoms and not a virus or bacteria. Prunes contain unusually high amounts of boron, and I have found they can cause breakouts, bloating, and queasiness, especially motion sickness, if I eat too many. Raisins, dates, avocados, almonds, peanuts, and other nuts can also contain significant amounts of boron.[50] I eat several of these foods on a regular basis and do not notice breakouts (perhaps it is a function of the co-factors?) but if you eat them in abundance, keep an eye out for signs of fluoride detoxification. Don't worry about memorizing this. It's all in the cheat sheet.[51]

Lesson #5: No Nutrient is an Island

Returning to the iodine angle, I finally got serious about learning the details of iodine supplementation and read *Iodine: Why You Need It, Why You Can't Live Without It* by David Brownstein, one of the Iodine Doctors. I also read *The Iodine Crisis* by Lynne Farrow, founder of Breast Cancer Choices. Both authors emphasize iodine supplementation as part of a complete nutritional program.

When fluoride is released back into circulation, your body needs extra nutrients to help eliminate it safely. I assumed that relying on nutrient-dense foods would be enough, but a healthy diet did not sufficiently counterbalance the effects of fluoride detoxification. A.K. Susheela, a fluoride researcher in India, uses essential nutrients and antioxidants to reverse the effects of skeletal fluorosis.[52] A traditional nutrient-dense diet is the best way to maintain good health but to overcome

---

[50] I considered the possibility that perhaps the toxic effect of raisins on dogs is caused by their boron content and not fluoride-based pesticides, but that theory did not fit in with other evidence such as the related fatalities from grapes, the lack of fatalities from other boron-rich foods, and the timing of the crimes. This is clearly a case of involuntary dogslaughter.

[51] To receive a copy of the cheat sheet, see **ProjectFree.Me/Fluoride.**

[52] Susheela, A.K.; Bhavnagar, Madhu. "Reversal of fluoride induced cell injury through elimination of fluoride and consumption of diet rich in essential nutrients and antioxidants," *Developments in Molecular and Cellular Biochemistry*, vol. 37, 2002, pp. 335-340.

fluoride poisoning, *an effective iodine supplementation program requires additional supplements including selenium, magnesium, vitamin C, and unrefined sea salt*. Selenium is particularly important. In the iodine supplementation plan developed by the Iodine Doctors, these supplements are referred to as companion nutrients.

Lesson #6: Little Things Add Up

When a job transfer took me to a new state, I finally lived within driving distance of one of the recommended "iodine-literate" doctors. I told him about my sensitivity to iodine and after ordering the necessary tests to check my thyroid gland, among other things, he helped me get started on the iodine program. I began with just the companion nutrients, building up to the recommended dosages over a period of a few weeks. I was also sensitive to selenium, so I began with a quarter of the recommended dose and added another quarter each week, reaching the full dose after one month.

After everything checked out with my blood tests, the doctor suggested I start iodine supplementation with one drop of Dulse Liquid which equates to 11 mcg of iodine. I added one drop per day until I reached the full dose of 225 mcg over a period of twenty days. I stayed there for two weeks before switching to a pill that contains 225 mcg of potassium iodide. In the past, this amount of iodine caused my skin to break out, but *because I started with a minuscule dose and added to it in small increments over a long period of time, I was able to increase my iodine intake with minimal side effects*. I took the potassium iodide pill for one week and then added another pill each week until I was taking 4 pills, or 900 mcg, of iodine per day.

Lesson #7: Good Help is Hard to Find

The doctor recommended I continue taking 4 iodine pills per day until I finish the bottle and then switch to Iodoral, the pill form of liquid Lugol's solution which was the iodine supplement of choice in the early twentieth century. Like Lugol's, Iodoral is a blend of potassium iodide and iodine. It is the supplement the Iodine Doctors use in their clinics since

Lugol's can irritate the stomach and the taste is repulsive to most people. The Iodoral tablet the doctor gave me was 12.5 mg, but he suggested I start with a half dose to see how my body reacted to it. My body reacted to it the same way it reacted to other large doses of iodine: acne, bloating, digestive problems and heart palpitations.

I tried cutting the pill in quarters and only taking it every other day, but it still did not go over well. I made an appointment with the doctor to discuss the difficulty I was having with Iodoral. He explained that some people just can't take larger doses of iodine and that I should stick to 900 mcg which is still a significant increase from what most people consume. I asked him about the iodine lab test I read about in Brownstein's book, and he did not seem to be familiar with it. If he was, he never bothered to order the test for me which led me to the conclusion that *even "iodine-literate" doctors might not be completely iodine-literate*.

Lesson #8: What You See Is Not All There Is

I first took the iodine-loading test in 2010 when Hakala Research Laboratory agreed to provide a free test kit in return for an article about it on my blog. At the time, I had healed my acne by avoiding fluoride, but it was before I figured out how to increase my consumption of iodine. The test involves taking a 50 mg iodine pill and then measuring the amount of iodine secreted in the urine for the next 24 hours. Working with their patients, the Iodine Doctors determined that iodine sufficiency is reached when the body eliminates 90 percent or more of the iodine pill within a 24-hour period. The test can also measure how much fluoride and bromide is excreted in this same timeframe.

According to my initial test results, my body eliminated 93 percent of the iodine pill. Hakala noted that a false high reading in your first test is a common result in people who have a "symporter defect" that causes iodine to not be properly absorbed by the cells. It typically resolves after several weeks of iodine supplementation. At 0.36 mg, my fluoride level was among the lowest they had ever seen which made sense since I had been avoiding fluoride for a couple years. But if my body was not eliminating fluoride, why was I having such a negative reaction from iodine? After I took the 50 mg pill, my skin broke out in a deep cystic welt but not until two days later. This fluoride would not have been captured in the 24-hour screening.

I have taken the iodine loading test multiple times in the last few years. As the lab predicted, my iodine results went down to 73 percent after I began taking a daily iodine supplement. But the fluoride measurements never gave an indication that a significant amount of fluoride was being released from my tissue. My bromide levels decreased from 16 mg to less than 3 mg as measured in the 24-hour urine screening, but after I started supplementing with iodine, the fluoride measurements stayed consistent at about 1 mg. I even ordered fluoride tests for the day before and several days after taking the 50 mg pill. My fluoride levels dipped slightly on the day the pill was taken but remained at 1.04 to 1.24 all the other days.

The Iodine Doctors seem to focus on bromide detoxification because that is what is reflected most in the 24-hour iodine loading test, but I suspect *the current testing methods are missing an important part of the fluoride picture*. Bromide has been widely found in fire retardants, pesticides, fumigants, and electronics as well as brominated flour used in baked goods and brominated vegetable oils used in Mountain Dew and other toxic beverages. Most Americans have been exposed to significant amounts of bromide, but it's not as if they add it to the water supply and guilt you into brushing your teeth with it twice a day.

*****

There are many potential explanations for why a sharp increase in fluoride is not measured in my 24-hour iodine loading test, but we are far from exploring them. We have barely begun to study these halogens, much less develop a deep understanding of all the intricate ways they interact with the human body.[53] The current medical research on halogens is oversimplified and unsophisticated. Most doctors still think fluoride's main effect is to prevent cavities. Studies don't differentiate between varying types of iodine. Seaweed is equated with iodine even though it contains many other chemical constituents, and the interaction of various goitrogens and important nutritional cofactors are almost completely neglected.

Reading over the history of iodine in the previous section, you might have noticed that current medical consensus is more a matter of the human story, not the science that scientists proclaim to have discovered. Who was promoted to a government soapbox? Whose studies support industry interests? Who died and stopped swaying scientific opinion in a certain direction or left behind a body of work unfinished? It will take a long time to develop a nuanced understanding of how these halogens affect the human body. If we want to be healthy now, we don't have time to wait for future generations to figure things out.

The Iodine Doctors put themselves at risk by incorporating iodine supplementation into their family practices while current medical opinion claims it is dangerous. They continue to do so because they have seen the dramatic positive effects iodine causes in their patients. Jan Wolff, on the other hand, spent his entire career dissecting rats in a laboratory. He worked with patients during his internship for medical school but didn't care for it.

In his 1969 review detailing the effect of excess iodine, Wolff references 280 scientific papers but he also notes, "The demonstration of the Wolff-Chaikoff effect in man remains presumptive." Scientists

---

[53] My main theory at the moment is that perhaps this situation is similar to the case when researchers at the Medical College of Georgia were unable to detect the level of fluoride they suspected was contained in instant tea that was causing skeletal fluorosis in several patients. When they developed a new diffusion method for testing the fluoride content of tea, they found much higher fluoride levels than when they used the traditional electrode method. The Iodine Doctors use the electrode method for measuring the fluoride content of urine. But who knows, there are many other possible explanations.

are not able to reproduce the Wolff-Chaikoff effect in the laboratory without the use of goitrogens. [54]

Like the Wright brothers and their airplane, the Iodine Doctors are at a great advantage in deciphering how the human body is affected by halogens because they are dealing with the human body directly in the physical world, not just in the abstract world of rat thyroids, lab tests, and scientific papers. We have that advantage, too.

Stuck at 900 mcg of iodine, I parted ways with the aforementioned "iodine-literate" doctor after he pulled an old doctor's tactic (you've probably seen this one before) where he sidesteps my questions by casually claiming they're nonsensical. The questions seemed perfectly unnonsensical to me, so I concluded it was time to move on. But how?

It was four years since I took my first kelp capsule, and I was still far from consuming the amount of iodine recommended by the Iodine Doctors. Was my doctor right, and some people just can't take iodine? My acne was gone and I felt healthy enough—was it worth pursuing further? I had researched the topic so much and experimented with iodine for so long that I felt like the answer was right in front me, but I couldn't quite make it out. I stopped reading about iodine. I stopped blogging. I gave up looking for a doctor who could show me the way. Instead, the way came to me.

I've been supplementing with 50 mg of iodine for almost eight months now. My iodine-loading test increased from 73 to 84 percent iodine saturation, and I am close to the 90 percent the Iodine Doctors note is correlated with optimal health. More importantly, the positive changes in my mind and body corroborate that I am on the right track. Before taking iodine, I came home from work exhausted. I thought being tired after work was normal, but now I have energy to do yoga, take a walk with my husband, go to dinner with a friend, play with

---

[54] Abraham, G.E., "The safe and effective implementation of orthoiodosupplementation in medical practice," The Original Internist, issue 11, 2004, pp. 17-36.

my dog, and generally live life outside of my 9 to 5 commitment.

The mental changes have been even greater. As someone who thinks for a living, I can attest that iodine caused a sharp increase in my mental acuity. I did not notice the fog until it lifted. To give just one example, I figured out fluoride causes acne several years ago and I knew it was not an uncommon condition, but I didn't realize the importance of writing this book until very recently. When it finally hit me, I didn't know if I would be able to write a whole book but here we are, four months and 72,000 words later.

I learned a lot about iodine from books, articles, doctors, and Internet, but for me, the key to effective iodine supplementation didn't come from any of those sources. It came from a bear on a mountaintop.

*****

Lions, Tigers, and a Bear

Scientific experiments are one way of learning about the world. Myths and stories are another. The following story is called "The Bear." It was passed down from Sgt. I. Sagara, a Japanese-American World War II veteran who was a patient at Hines Veteran's Assistance Hospital in Illinois many moons ago. He happened to tell the tale to Clarissa Pinkola Estes, a Jungian psychoanalyst and *cantadora*, keeper of the old stories.

For anyone struggling with detoxification, whether the offending matter is emotional or physical, the wisdom revealed in "The Bear" shows how to proceed. Clarissa passed this story along to me in her brilliant bestselling book, *Women Who Run With the Wolves: Myths and Stories of the Wild Woman Archetype.*[55] I will retell it for you here in my own words and then we can sift over the secrets it contains.

---

[55] Read it!

*****

*Once there was, and once there was not,[56] a young woman who
lived in a fragrant pine forest in the islands of Japan. She loved to
explore her small island and converse with the mountains and
streams, while her husband was content to view the mountains
from their front porch and to sip his tea. They were very happy
together. One day, the husband was sent off to war. When he
returned many years later, he no longer enjoyed sipping his tea on
the front porch and refused to enter the house, instead sleeping
outside on a pile of stones as he had done during the war.*

*Nevertheless, the young wife was overjoyed to have her husband
returned to her. She cooked for him the most magnificent meals she
could cook. Small fishes and large fishes. Small shrimps and large
shrimps. Bowls overflowing with rice and fermented bean curd.
Five kinds of seaweed. But when she delivered the tray of food to her
husband, he knocked it to the ground and warned her to leave him
be. Knowing he was hungry, she tried again and again but was met
with the same response. After many failed attempts, the woman
consulted the wise healer who lived in a cave on the outskirts of
their village. The healer told her she would need a special ingredient
to remedy her husband's rage—a silver hair from the chest of the
black bear known to inhabit a nearby mountaintop.*

*The young wife was relieved that a cure for her husband was within
reach. She took to the mountain undaunted by the task ahead,
calling out "Arigato zaisho" to thank it for allowing her to climb its
steep boulders. When tree limbs blocked her path, again she called
out "Arigato zaisho" as a way to thank them for allowing her to
pass underneath. In the evening, when dark birds flew at her head,
she recognized them as the spirits of dead ancestors who were not
properly laid to rest. She prayed for them and blessed them as she
ascended to the mountain's peak.*

*Finally, the woman reached the den of the black bear where she
could hear his weighted breath inside. Reaching into her pack, she*

---

[56] As Clarissa explains, this opening phrase is one of the oldest storytelling devices.
She didn't use it in her version of "The Bear," but I chose to include it in mine.
According to Clarissa, "This paradoxical phrase is meant to alert the soul of the
listener that this story takes place in the world between worlds where nothing is as it
first seems."

pulled out a bowl of the food she prepared for her husband. She left it by the entrance to the cave and then ran off to hide in the forest. When the aroma of her cooking reached the bear's nostrils, he arose from his dirt bed and waited at the edge of his den, scanning the air for signs of danger. Finding none, he reached down into the bowl and swallowed the whole meal in one toothy bite.

Each evening, the woman left a bowl of food this way for the black bear, but instead of hiding in the forest, she inched her way closer so the bear's nostrils would grow accustomed to her scent. One night, as the bear was just about to clamp his jaws shut and devour his complimentary dinner, he noticed a small pair of human feet enter the clearing in front of him. Startled, he shook his head, roared, and railed back on his hind legs until he was taller than the tallest point of the mountain. The woman trembled but she did not run.

"Please don't hurt me," the woman said. "I've been feeding you all these nights in the hope that you will give me a silver hair from your chest so I can use it to cure my dear husband." The bear slowly returned his front paws to the earth. When he looked deep into the woman's eyes and saw nothing but love for her husband, he knew she was being truthful. The bear lifted his head and allowed the woman to pluck a single silver hair from the white V across his chest. Then he roared at her to leave and never return.

The woman ran all the way back down the mountain, crying "Arigato zaisho" to the trees and birds and boulders as she passed.

*****

Can you hear Mr. Sagara telling Clarissa this tale from his bed in the veteran's hospital, the images of war still vivid in his mind's eye? Clarissa explains "The Bear" as a story about emotional healing but it is just as fitting to describe it as a story about physical healing. Like rage, when we discover our bodies are hardened with fluoride we want to hurry up and get rid of it. "It is a little like toxic waste," Clarissa says. "There it is, no one wants it, but there are few disposal areas for it. One has to travel far in order to find a burial ground."

As in virtually all the myths Clarissa recounts, the various characters in "The Bear" are components of an individual woman's psyche. The wife is the loving aspect, the husband is the injured part, and the healer is the wisest self. "Healers in fairy tales generally represent a calm and unperturbed aspect of the psyche," Clarissa tells us. "Even though the world may be falling to pieces outwardly, the inner healer is unswayed by it all and maintains the calm to figure out the best way to proceed. Every woman's psyche contains this 'fixer.' It is part of the wild and natural psyche and we are born with it." This is the healer I called on to heal from fluoride, and you are free to call on her, too.

Like the wife's journey on the mountain, the journey to rid your body of fluoride might be long and wrought with stumbling blocks. But if these obstacles are approached with the right attitude, they can be an important part of the healing process. Clarissa points out that the tree limbs represent the lifting of our illusions. What illusions might you have with fluoride? Are you under the impression that your body will never be healthier than it is today? That disease is inevitable? That only doctors can heal?

The dark birds that fly at the wife's head are other injured parts of her psyche that are released as she climbs the mountain. She does not shoo them away but instead cares for them and comforts them with her prayers. These birds are like the negative side effects people experience when they detoxify with iodine. Skin rashes, a metallic taste in your mouth, bloating and digestive difficulties, fatigue—these side effects are not to be ignored or shooed away, but tended to as you would care for a loved one. Maybe you need to reduce your dose of iodine for a while or take a few days off. Maybe your body needs extra sleep or extra nutrients. An extra long salt bath, extra sunshine, or extra love.

When it comes to ridding your body of fluoride, the woman's interaction with the black bear teaches us the most important lesson of all. It takes time to draw the bear out of his cave. You have to feed him slowly, inching your way closer every day without any sudden movements. The doctor wanted me to jump from 900 mcg of iodine to 6 mg in a single day. This leap frightened the bear and left me running down the mountain empty-handed. When I made my way back to its summit, I decided I would be patient this time, and I continued to increase the amount of iodine by micro-increments. Instead of jumping to 6 mg, I increased to 1, then 1.2 a few days later, then 1.4 and so on.[57] It took a solid year before I finally looked the bear in the eyes and pulled the silver hair from his chest.

Like rage, fluoride can be a teacher for a time. It can teach you how to listen to your body. It can teach you how to care for yourself when your self needs caring for. As the story of "The Bear" illustrates, it can be a reason to climb the mountain.

I am not under the delusion that my way of detoxifying from fluoride is the final way or the best way. It is possible that boron or cilantro or fairy dust is more effective and causes fewer side effects. And certainly, there are secrets to iodine still to be uncovered. We are only at the beginning stages of understanding halogens, but there is another reason I believe iodine is the key to unlocking the whole mystery. *Hal-* is a word-forming element from Greek meaning *salt* or *sea*. *-Gen* signifies *giving birth to*. In its most basic sense, the term halogen conveys the idea of giving birth to the sea. What a provocative notion considering the sea is what gave birth to all life as we know it.

As you can probably tell, there's a story here. When I started digging into the topic of iodine for this book, I stumbled across the answer to a question humans have been asking since the early days of humans asking questions. The story explains why iodine is critical for healthy skin. But it also explains a lot more than that.

*****

---

[57] Visit **ProjectFree.Me/Iodine** for my 1-page Quick Guide on my experience detoxifying fluoride with iodine.

In The Beginning

*"We shall not cease from exploration,
and the end of all our exploring will be to arrive where we started
and know the place for the first time."*

—T.S. Elliott

Analysis of intelligence failures reveal they are more commonly caused by flawed assumptions rather than flawed information. Relying on assumptions in analysis is unavoidable. Instead of trying to avoid assumptions, intelligence analysts are encouraged to try to make their assumptions as explicit as possible, stating them up front so they can be challenged and if appropriate, disconfirmed. Assumptions that have the greatest impact on an assessment are called lynchpin assumptions. Challenging lynchpin assumptions is a valuable technique in moving an assessment forward.

It is not surprising that the government-sanctioned mainstream medical community is confused about the daily requirement for iodine, so I won't bother challenging their assumptions that government-approved drugs are the answer to everything and that diet is for dummies. But the alternative health community, for lack of a better term, is generally in agreement that nutrition is the key to health and that fluoride is a neurotoxin that depresses thyroid function. Yet many alternative health advocates are wary to endorse the milligram amounts of iodine that the Iodine Doctors claim are correlated with optimal health in their patients.

Here is a typical conversation about iodine from one of my favorite paleo bloggers, Stephan Guyenet, that illustrates a lynchpin assumption of why milligram doses of iodine are not widely endorsed by the alternative health community. (I'm pointing at the lynchpin *like this.*)

> **Tom writes at "Iodine" on WholeHealthSource:**[58] Stephan, any opinion on the merit of high-dose iodine therapy as advocated by Guy Abraham and David Brownstein?
>
> > **Gunther Gatherer replies:** Those two doctors prescribe Iodoral at 12.5 mg iodine per tablet, and claim therapeutic effects at doses of even up to a gram daily. *Just doesn't seem very paleo to me*... BTW Stephen, don't eggs contain a fair amount? So any paleo diet approach containing them should cover us, no?
> >
> > **Stephan Guyenet replies:** Tom, I don't know but *anything outside of a natural range of intake makes me suspicious*... Gunther, eggs do seem to be a good source. As with dairy, the amount will depend on what the animals are eating. In the midwest, dairy and eggs didn't keep them from getting goiter before iodized salt because the soil is deficient.

One of the assumptions both Gunther and Stephan make in their reply to Tom is that the traditional homo sapien diet is an important guide for how we should eat today. Even though we are likely exposed to more toxic sources of fluoride and other goitrogens, I largely support that assumption, so I'm not going to challenge it here. Another assumption they both make is that milligram amounts of iodine are not native to the homo sapien diet. That's the one I am going to challenge. We are about to cover a lot of ground, so be sure to keep up. Here we go.

There are a number of techniques that can be used to challenge assumptions. The one I am choosing to use here is called "thinking backwards," also referred to as the "crystal ball" technique. Thinking backwards is an intellectual exercise that begins with an assumption

---

[58] Comments posted at "Iodine" by Stephen Guyenet at WholeHealthSource. blogspot.com , May 2, 2009 (available at http://wholehealthsource.blogspot.com/ 2009/05/iodine.html).

contrary to the assumption you are challenging. For example, say you make an assumption that penguins are not capable of producing a nuclear weapon. In the thinking backwards exercise, you start with the assumption that penguins *are* capable of producing a nuclear weapon and then you think backwards to figure out what events had to occur a year ago (or a million years ago) to make that happen. It's as if you looked into a crystal ball and saw that in the near future penguins do in fact detonate an atomic bomb. *Surprise!* Now your job as an analyst is to go back and put the pieces together that you missed the first time around.

By imagining an unexpected future event, you are forcing yourself to see the current situation differently. As Heuer explains in *Psychology of Intelligence Analysis*, "Analysts will often find, to their surprise, that they can construct a quite plausible scenario for an event they had previously thought unlikely… This suggests your assumption is open to some question."

In our scenario, we look into the crystal ball and see that enlightened paleo dieters of the future conclude beyond question that daily milligram doses of iodine are—and always have been—a natural part of a healthy homo sapien diet. How did we miss that? We need to go back and put the pieces together. Starting with the present day, we now challenge ourselves to think backwards over time to figure out how humans could have become dependent on milligram doses of iodine.

If we are looking for evidence of significant consumption of iodine in a healthy human diet, we are not likely to find it in present-day populations. The current global prevalence of inadequate iodine consumption is widely recognized. The World Health Organization claims two billion people consume less than 100 micrograms of iodine per day, making iodine deficiency the single greatest cause of intellectual disability.[59] Researchers from *The Lancet* estimate that 187

---

[59] de Benoist, Bruno et. al. "Iodine deficiency in 2007: Global progress since 2003," *Food and Nutrition Bulletin*, vol 29, issue 3, 2008.

million people suffer from goiter due to a lack of dietary iodine, approximately 2.7 percent of the global population.[60] Even cretinism, now referred to as congenital hypothyroidism, has been found to be on the rise in the last two decades in the United States, although it is now reversible when detected in early screenings.[61]

To expand our search, a more fruitful approach is to study societies where global food corporations like Nestle and Coca-Cola have yet to make their mark. Such societies are difficult to find today but less than one hundred years ago that was not the case. Furthermore, we don't want to throw a dart at the map and study any non-industrialized society—we want to find the healthiest ones and focus on those.

This next sentence might come as a shock. The best research I've found detailing the traditional diets of the healthiest human societies in the world came from a dentist. (*I know, right?!*) His name was Weston Price, and he travelled the world in the 1930s looking for societies where tooth decay was rare. He found groups of people in Europe, Africa, Asia, Australia, and the Americas who displayed a remarkably high resistance to dental decay. But what was even more astonishing was that these same societies also seemed to be resistant to many of the health disorders plaguing the industrialized world, from tuberculosis and heart failure to cancer and varicose veins. Price concluded that dental decay is a symptom of deeper health problems caused by poor nutrition.

In his book published in 1939, *Nutrition and Physical Degeneration*, Price describes his travels to these societies and includes details of their traditional diets. He also includes photographs to demonstrate the dietary traditions that produce strong teeth, as well as

---

[60] Cos, Theo et. al. "Years lived with disability (YLDs) for 1160 sequelae of 289 diseases and injuries 1990–2010: a systematic analysis for the Global Burden of Disease Study 2010," *The Lancet*, vol. 380, issue 9859, Dec 2012, pp. 2163–2196.

[61] Olney, Richard S., et. al. "Prevalence of Congenital Hypothyroidism—Current Trends and Future Directions: Workshop Summary," *Pediatrics*, vol. 125, issue 2, May 2010.

the deleterious effects that result when native people switch to a diet of sugar, flour, and other modern foods. His book is compelling evidence that traditional diets are an effective way to prevent the so-called "diseases of civilization." But what can it tell us about iodine? If our crystal ball is correct, and for this exercise we must assume it is, then these healthy societies must have been consuming high amounts of iodine. Now it's our job to figure out how they could have done it.

Most of the groups Price describes in his book consume copious amounts of seafood. Traditional Polynesians, Melanesians, Aborigines, Eskimos, Gaelics, Native American Indians, New Zealand Maori, and Torres Straight Islanders all lived predominantly off the sea. Eskimos fed their children fish eggs as their first food after weaning and developed complex processes to turn kelp into dried cakes that could be stored and eaten during winter.[62] Pacific Islanders put an emphasis on shellfish and made great efforts to collect them in abundance, also eating a variety of seaweed as part of their regular diet. On the west coast of Scotland, a seaweed called dulce was eaten in a thick broth with oats or simply boiled and served with butter. Other types of seaweed were turned into sauces, soups, and puddings.

So many of the healthy societies Price encountered relied on seafood that he deliberately embarked on arduous travel inland in the hopes of finding people without cavities who did not include food from the sea in their diet. He did not always succeed. When he visited Viti Levu, for example, the largest island in Fiji, he drove deep into the interior and then proceeded on foot but was disappointed by the piles of seashells that lined the path. His guide informed him that even during times of bitter warfare, the inland people found a way to trade with coastal rivals for essential foods from the sea. Several of Price's guides in the Pacific islands revealed that a lack of essential seafoods for people living in the interior was the primary motivation for

---

[62] Kuhnlein, Harriet V.; Turner, Nancy K. "Traditional Plant Foods of Canadian Indigenous Peoples: Nutrition, Botany and Use," Gordon and Breach Publishers, 1991.

cannibalism. It was common knowledge that fisherman were "especially sought for staying a famine" because of the nutrients from the sea their bodies contained.[63]

During his years of travel, Price does manage to find a few healthy societies who do not eat seafood. These are the groups that paleo dieters and traditional food enthusiasts use to demonstrate that the amount of iodine recommended by the Iodine Doctors is not a normal part of the homo sapien diet. But since our crystal ball already told us that these doses of iodine *are* required for optimal health, our challenge in this exercise is to figure out how these people could have obtained iodine without consuming food from the sea.

Next to seafood, the other major food group Price identifies as preventing dental decay is dairy. Is it a coincidence that next to seafood, the other major food source of iodine is dairy? Unlike fluoride, iodine is eagerly passed on to babies through mother's milk.

The best example from Price's book comes from the residents of a town in the Swiss Alps where the diet consisted largely of dairy products, rye bread, meat once a week, and some vegetables in the summer. Milk doesn't contain nearly as much iodine as seaweed, but the people Price encountered in the Swiss valley weren't your average milk drinkers. They were a little obsessed with it. Not only were dairy products their primary source of calories—a bowl of heavy cream was considered the quintessential health beverage—but they literally celebrated the presence of divinity in the June butter produced from cows grazing near the snow line in summer. (The ceremony involved lighting a wick in a bowl of butter and letting it burn in a special sanctuary, as one does.)

Early in Price's book, he comments that people previously believed a lack of iodine was the cause of the rampant dental decay in Switzerland, but he quickly dismisses this possibility. As Price

---

[63] Price, Weston A., "Studies of Relationships Between Nutritional Deficiencies and (a) Facial and Dental Arch Deformities and (b) Loss of Immunity to Dental Caries Among South Sea Islanders and Florida Indians." *The Dental Cosmos.* 77(11), 1935, pp. 1033-45.

explains, "That this is not the case seems clearly demonstrated by the fact that dental caries is apparently as extensive today as before, if not more so, while the iodine problem has been met through a reinforcement of the diet of growing children and others in stress periods with iodine in suitable form." *But Wes, what if iodized salt is only sufficient for preventing goiter and cretinism but not dental decay and other signs of physical degeneration?* He doesn't seem to consider that possibility. Later in the book, Price writes about the inadequacy of reinforcing the diet with a few synthetic products known to represent certain nutrients, but he never applies this point of view to iodized salt. Dentists are so weird.

The Masai people in Africa are another group of dairy enthusiasts Price identifies as prime examples of robust health. They are even more serious about their cows than the Swiss group. When it comes to livestock, the Masai would be considered a little on the OCD side by our current standards. As Price explains, they carefully cultivate their herd by judging their cows on how quickly a calf starts running after it is born, which for a Masai calf is only a matter of minutes. The Masai's primary diet consists of milk, meat, blood, and a few vegetables. When available, growing children and pregnant or lactating mothers receive a daily ration of raw blood. The iodine content of Masai cow blood is difficult to track down but where there is thyroid hormone, there is iodine. Could blood have been the extra source of iodine that gave the Masai people their physical prowess?

The farther Price moved from the sea, the more resourceful and creative the people he studied seem to become with their diets. The Native American Indians of northern British Columbia and Yukon Territory were some of the most remote societies he visited. They did not have access to seafood, not even migrating salmon, and it was too cold for dairy or agriculture. Instead, they lived predominantly off wild game such as moose and caribou. This is the group Sally Fallon Morrell, President of the Weston Price Foundation, points to in her article, "The Great Iodine Debate," when she asserts that the amount of iodine consumed by the people Price studied is mostly in line with the current Recommended Daily Allowance.[64] But our crystal ball already told us that the people in these healthy societies must be getting a hefty dose of iodine from somewhere. Does Price provide any clues as to where?

In his book, Price notes that the Inuit of the far North live mostly off the organ meats of wild game, not the muscle meat as we prefer today. He even remarks on their ability to select certain organ meats and tissues to prevent specific diseases. At one point, he asks an older man in the group why his people do not suffer from scurvy, a disease caused by a lack of vitamin C. At first, the man says it is simply a white man's disease (the ol' genetic argument—heard that one before) but after asking for permission from the chief, he tells Price their secret. When a family consumes a moose, they divide the two small balls above the kidneys so that each family member is given a share. These are the moose's adrenal glands and as Price points out, they are the richest source of vitamin C in all animal or plant tissues.

What secret would the man have revealed if Price had asked about goiter? Do they also consume the moose's thyroid gland? Do caribou, like cows, have an iodine recycling system in their oral-salivary and gastro-intestinal tract to protect them against low dietary iodine?[65] If the Inuit ate these organs, how much iodine would they consume? The Inuit scrape every last morsel of bone marrow and emphasize its value for growing children. Does iodine, like fluoride,

---

[64] I could not find evidence to support the ranges of iodine Fallon says Price reported in the diets of Inuit and Eskimos. The reference she provides is a personal communication with Anore Jones, author of *Fish That We Eat*, a report on the diet of the Inupiat people in Northern Alaska. Despite claiming Price measured a range of iodine intake under 200 mcg per day for Inuit and Eskimos, Jones' 290-page report on the Inupiat diet contains 374 references to fish eggs. Fallon also forgets to include all the sea-bordering societies of the Pacific on the list of groups Price found who consume seaweed, instead highlighting only the Gaelics and some American Indians. SOURCE: Fallon Morrell, Sally. "The Great Iodine Debate," The Weston A. Price Foundation, Jun 22, 2009.

[65] Venturi, Sebastian. "Evolutionary Significance of Iodine," *Current Chemical Biology*, vol. 5, issue 3, 2011.

accumulate in bone? Or, is it possible the Inuit traded with coastal groups for dried kelp, as northern groups in British Columbia were known to do?[66]

Other inland groups were equally as resourceful. In Africa, they made ant pies, mayfly pudding, and a type of flour from dried locusts. Price notes, "the natives of Africa know that certain insects are very rich in special food values at certain seasons, also that their eggs are valuable foods." Did inland Africans select their insects based on their iodine content, like the inland people of Taxco, Mexico do with stinkbugs?[67] Insect eggs were especially valued. Is it a coincidence that next to seafood and milk, eggs are known as a significant source of iodine? Inland Aborigines and Amazon Indians also included eggs in their diet whenever possible, particularly eggs from waterfowl and other birds. In the high Andes of Peru, Price found that people travelled hundreds of miles to gather fish eggs so they would not get "big neck" like the white people do. Dried kelp was equally important.

Because of the Humboldt Current and the extraordinary array of marine life it brings to the coast of Peru, Price was particularly interested in the ancient people who lived along the western coast of South America. In a study of 1,276 skeletal remains, he did not find a single deformity of the dental arches. Price laments that little is known about the ancient cultures that lived there, but he does tell us their modern counterparts emphasize the importance of fish eggs for the development of children, especially girls. The glands of a certain fish, the angelote, were consumed by young couples prior to conceiving. Weighing up to a pound each when dried, the male glands were a special food eaten by fathers-to-be to ensure healthy offspring.

Despite the large amount of fish eggs and seaweed Price encounters in his travels, he overlooks the importance of iodine which

[66] Kuhnlein, Harriet V.; Turner, Nancy K. "Traditional Plant Foods of Canadian Indigenous Peoples: Nutrition, Botany and Use," Gordon and Breach Publishers, 1991.

[67] Sala, Mike. "Stinkbug salsa for the iodine deficient," *The Chicago Reader*, Oct 14, 2013.

he sees as a trace mineral the human body only requires in minute quantities. Instead, he attributes robust health primarily to large amounts of fat-soluble vitamins.[68] Price allows for much more sophistication in his conception of vitamins than with minerals, but iodine isn't exactly a vitamin or a mineral. As we discussed in chapter three, it is a halogen.

Furthermore, it would take enormous effort to calculate the iodine content of the traditional diets Price studied to quantify their true values. Not only is it difficult to determine the iodine content of mayflies during a designated period in their mating season, but as we have seen time after time, the nutritional content of a specific food depends on a myriad of factors, making an established average little more than a vague suggestion.

For the average American, it might not be considered normal to consume milligrams of iodine, but clearly "normal" is a matter of perspective. In most of the groups Price studied, the seaweed and fish eggs in their diet could easily provide daily doses of iodine in the milligram amounts. For the inland groups, it is possible their meticulous diets were intentionally constructed to be rich in iodine from dairy products, select organ meats, eggs, and other unconventional sources.

Continuing our thinking backwards exercise, what about the first people in the Americas? Weren't they savage nomads running around spearing mammoths and mastodons? Price admits to knowing very little about the culture of the ancient people of South America. So did modern anthropologists until 1975 when a local farmer in a region of southern Chile called Monte Verde found a strange "cow bone" and showed it to a visiting veterinary student. The bone turned out to be from a mastodon, and it dramatically altered the prevailing view of the early peoples of the Americas.

---

[68] I'm not saying his assessment is inaccurate, but I am saying that if our crystal ball turns out to be telling us the truth, then his analysis wrongfully neglects iodine and needs to be reworked in light of new information.

It is difficult for archeologists to reconstruct a full picture of evolutionary diets from the bits of stone, bone and teeth that remain in ancient ruins, but the Monte Verde site was special. When archaeologists excavated the region where the mastodon bone was found, they uncovered the remains of an ancient community that lived along the banks of Chinchihuapi Creek located 36 miles from the current Pacific coastline. Shortly after the region was originally occupied, the waters of the creek rose to form a peat-filled bog that inhibited the bacterial decay of organic material left at the site, preserving perishable artifacts for millennia.

What did archaeologists find amongst the wooden tools, scraps of leather, human footprints and chunks of mastodon meat? Nine species of seaweed, along with a type of algae that grows exclusively on littoral rocks and trees. The seaweed was collected across a variety of regions and seasons. Because of its widespread dispersion in hearths and cooking areas throughout the site, archaeologists concluded it was used for both food and medicinal purposes. All nine species were found to be an excellent source of iodine.[69]

There is another aspect of the Monte Verde site that made it special. Not only is it one of the rare open-air prehistoric communities found in the Americas, but when archaeologists dated the site they determined it is 14,800 years old—over a millennia older than the oldest known settlement in the Americas at the time. Many experts refused to accept the age of the Monte Verde site because they had already created a nice story depicting the first homo sapiens crossing into the Americas after the retreating ice age opened the Bering land bridge from Siberia to Alaska 13,000 years ago. How could a band of homo sapiens have settled in the southern tip of Chile 1,800 years *before* the land bridge opened?

Forced to reconsider their theory, some archaeologists proposed it was a coastal migration that brought homo sapiens from

---

[69] Dillehay, Tom D., et. al. "Monte Verde: Seaweed, Food, Medicine, and the Peopling of South America," *Science,* vol. 320, issue 5877, May 9, 2008, pp. 784-786.

Asia to the Americas. Instead of trekking to the New World across a land bridge on foot, they believe people sailed along the coast and quickly migrated all the way to the southern tip of South America by boat.

The coastal migration theory was a major departure from the previous view, but it steadily gained support as evidence mounted. Another important clue was unearthed in the mid-1990s when paleontologists were excavating an ancient bear den on the tip of Prince of Wales Island in southeastern Alaska. Contrary to previous views that these island chains were covered in glacial ice during the last ice age and uninhabitable, researchers uncovered animal remains indicating the cave was continuously inhabited for the past 40,000 years. Then in 1996, they found the bones of a 10,000-year-old homo sapien, the oldest human remains ever found in Alaska or Canada.

Even though the man's bones were found 300 miles inland where land meats were abundant, isotopic analysis revealed they have the signature of a seal or ocean fish, meaning the man's diet was almost exclusively from the sea. Stone tools made of a volcanic glass called obsidian were also found at the site. Archeologists conclude it was likely brought in by boat from Mount Edziza in British Columbia 150 miles away. The man's mitochondrial DNA matched 47 samples from American Indians located down the western coast of the Americas, further supporting the idea of a rapid coastal expansion.

What started as a fringe theory in the 1970s went mainstream by 2007 when Jon Erlandson from the University of Oregon published his article, "The Kelp Highway Hypothesis."[70] Erlandson proposed that seafaring homo sapiens followed a linear progression of dense kelp forests that lined the coast from Japan to Alaska to the southern point of California and then resumed along the Andean Coast from Peru to Tierra del Fuego.

---

[70] Erlandson, Jon M. et. al. "The Kelp Highway Hypothesis: Marine Ecology, the Coastal Migration Theory, and the Peopling of the Americas," *The Journal of Island and Coastal Archaeology*, vol. 2, issue 2, 2001, pp. 161-174.

Kelp forests are known to support complex food webs in coastal ecosystems. Such ecosystems are relatively homogenous and would have made it easier for migrating peoples to adapt to new territory as long as they followed the coastline. Kelp, fish, and shellfish are familiar foods to both an Eskimo in Alaska and an American Indian on the coast of Peru.

In a land migration, on the other hand, people would have encountered a variety of unfamiliar physical barriers and terrestrial ecosystems, from Arctic tundra to woodland forests, grasslands and deserts. The animal and plant life varies widely in these landscapes, and it would have taken migrating people longer to figure out how to survive in their new environment. Erlandson also points out that some of the earliest settlements in North America are located adjacent to kelp forests, although the majority of the archaeological record of the kelp highway is most likely lost since ancient shorelines were buried under rising seas when the glaciers melted.

Homo sapiens already proved themselves to be expert navigators by this time, having been the only hominid species to reach Australia and other remote island groups roughly 50,000 years ago. Some of these islands were separated by over a hundred miles of open water and yet there is evidence of early trade routes in the region, particularly for obsidian, the volcanic glass used to make stone tools.[71] The peopling of the Australian continent was even more impressive given the terrestrial life there was unlike anything sapiens would have ever seen before. Giant marsupials dominated the landscape, from multi-ton wombats to 400-pound kangaroos and marsupial lions. Still, it is likely the earliest human visitors had little trouble finding something to eat. Kelp, fish, and shellfish are familiar foods to both an Eskimo in Alaska and a homo sapien on the coast of Australia.

In addition to Erlandon's Kelp Highway Hypothesis for explaining how homo sapiens arrived in the Americas, anthropologists

---

[71] Harari, Yuval Noah. *Sapiens: A Brief History of Humankind*. New York: HarperCollins Publishers, 2015.

also use a coastal migration theory to explain the rapid expansion of homo sapiens out of Africa, tracing a route to the Arabian Peninsula and then India, Southeast Asia, coastal China, Japan, New Guinea, Australia, and Oceania. Studies of genetics and linguistics support their theory. Even Weston Price on his visit to Africa commented on the similarity between the Ethiopians and the Polynesians he studied the previous year in the South Pacific, noting commonalities between certain words in their respective languages.

So here we are, on the shores of ancient Africa in our thinking backwards exercise. We traced the route of our sapien ancestors along a kelp highway from the mountains of Peru to the waters of the Pacific and then west to the birthplace of humanity. Surely this is where our hunt for milligram doses of iodine in the human diet must end, is it not?

The trail appears to go cold. Hominid predecessors in Africa were chimpanzees who evolved climbing trees and making funny banana jokes. They didn't eat seafood or drink milk. Their diet doesn't seem to hinge on the inclusion of eggs, blood, or organ meats. Archaeologists are *all kinds* of confused about how homo sapiens happened. They appear to spend a lot of time arguing over what they should name things and generally rely on the theory of natural selection to skirt around more useful questions like why exactly did homo sapiens go on to populate the planet (not *how*, that's a different story).

But archaeologists do have a theory on why early sapiens decided to live at the beach. During the second to last ice age, which started roughly 200,000 years ago, climate change in Africa turned rain forests and grasslands into desert. Some hominids like homo erectus and homo neanderthalensis had already made their way out of Africa by this time, but the hominids who would go on to become sapiens remained on the continent where they were pushed to the brink of extinction. DNA analysis reveals lower than expected genetic variation in present-day humans, which anthropologists attribute to a dramatic population crash in early homo sapiens.[72] It is possible the number of breeding individuals dwindled to a thousand or even fewer.

When Curtis Marean learned about the population bottleneck that geneticists were studying in the early 1990s, he was an archaeologist in East Africa's "cradle of humanity" studying the origin of modern humans. Marean began analyzing geologic formations, sea currents, and climate data to pinpoint a non-desertified region in Africa where early homo sapiens could have survived the climatic upheaval caused by Marine Isotope Stage 6. His analysis led to the caves of South Africa where dropping ocean levels during the ice age would have revealed a slope of the continental shelf rich in marine life that washed in with the tides. In 1999, he identified a series of caves on a promontory that juts into the Indian Ocean as a promising place to start looking for evidence of early homo sapiens. The spot is known as Pinnacle Point, and it proved to be hiding plenty of secrets Marean and his colleagues were about to uncover.

The excavations that followed unearthed a record of the homo sapiens who lived along the coast of South Africa between 164,000 and 35,000 years ago, the timeframe immediately after the bottleneck while the population was starting to recover. In 2007 Marean published his initial results in an article in *Nature* documenting that Pinnacle Point revealed the earliest known human use of marine resources and coastal habitats.[73] Homo sapiens were consuming shellfish there as early as 164,000 years ago. This was a radical change from the terrestrial plants and animals that hominids had been consuming for millions of years.

But seafood was only the beginning of the revolutionary finds uncovered at Pinnacle Point. In 2009, Marean published another breakthrough in the journal *Science* demonstrating that heat-treated

---

[72] Marean, Curtis W. "When the Sea Saved Humanity," *Scientific American*, Aug 2010.

[73] Marean, Curtis W. et. al. "Early human use of marine resources and pigment in South Africa during the Middle Pleistocene," *Nature*, vol. 449, Oct 18, 2007, pp. 905-908.

stone tools were already a dominant technology among homo sapiens 71,000 years ago.[74] Researchers previously believed the technology was invented in France just 20,000 years ago, but evidence from Pinnacle Point shows their conclusion was off by 50,000 years.

Early homo sapiens in South Africa even used microlithic technology, small bladelets of heat-treated stones used to create advanced projectile weapons.[75] The team also discovered dozens of pieces of red ochre at the site which showed signs they were ground into a powder and used as pigment. Marean argues this red ochre is the earliest unequivocal example of symbolic behavior. His research suggests that paleoanthropologists had been grossly underestimating the cognitive capabilities of early homo sapiens.

The results of Marean's excavations at Pinnacle Point were published in a cover story in *Scientific American* entitled, "When the Sea Saved Humanity."[76] In the article, Marean hypothesizes that homo sapiens who migrated south to the sea during Marine Isotope Stage 6 thrived on the unique combination of plant and animal life in the famous Cape Floral Region of South Africa, an area that contains the highest diversity of flora for its size anywhere in the world. By studying the type of shells found in layers of sediment at the site, researchers were able to determine when the inhabitants figured out how to collect shellfish from deeper intertidal zones, indicating that 110,000 years ago, people scheduled their trips to the shore based on their observations of lunar effects on the tides.

In addition to shellfish, Marean also emphasizes the importance of geophytes in the early homo sapien diet. Geophytes are high-carbohydrate underground bulbs and tubers that Marean

---

[74] Brown, K.S.; Marean, C.W., et. al. "Fire as an engineering tool of early modern humans," *Science*, vol. 325, issue 5942, Aug 14, 2009, pp. 859-862.

[75] Brown, K.S.; Marean, C.W., et. al., "An early and enduring advanced technology originating 71,000 years ago in South Africa," *Nature*, vol. 491, Nov 22, 2012, pp. 590-593.

[76] Marean, Curtis W. "When the Sea Saved Humanity," *Scientific American*, Aug 2010.

speculates early humans relied on as an easy source of dietary energy. His team did not uncover any evidence of geophyte consumption, however, which is not surprising since ancient organic matter is rarely preserved. Marean neglects to consider seaweed as an important factor in the evolution of modern humans, yet it is not difficult to imagine it being one of the first seafoods that sapiens tasted. When humans first stepped onto the beach, why *wouldn't* they eat the edible plants the sea literally dropped at their feet with each new wave?

The story of modern humans is a story about returning to the sea. Prior to our exile from the African interior, early sapiens were on the same evolutionary trajectile as other hominids. Our relatives from the homo genus were an intelligent group. Homo erectus occupied Eurasia for well over a million years, making it the most enduring human species to ever walk the planet. Yet there is no indication they ever ventured to the shores of Australia. They were skilled hunters and are believed to be among the first hominids to use controlled fire, but their stone technology was relatively unchanged throughout their existence. Sapien teenagers would never stand for that.

What made homo erectus and homo sapiens so different that one lived for nearly two million years as a relatively low-impact predator on the Eurasian landmass while the other exploded out of Africa roughly 100,000 years ago and quickly travelled to the farthest ends of the earth and beyond, altering everything in its path?

The experts speculate a variety of reasons for why homo sapiens turned out to be such a dominant species—it is because we make complex tools, we learned how to hunt by throwing things, we trade food for sex, we're highly social.[77] But these explanations leave us largely unsatisfied because they are tautological. They are more a description of *how* humans behave rather than an explanation of *why* we came to behave this way.

---

[77] For several unsatisfying explanations and an equally unsatisfying explanation of why all the explanations are unsatisfying, see http://news.nationalgeographic.com/2015/09/150911-how-we-became-human-theories-evolution-science/.

The caves at Pinnacle Point are still being excavated and probably have many more secrets to tell, along with archaeological sites in the region yet to be discovered. But the most exciting find isn't the bits of shells and stones left at the site. Marean suggests that passing down complex processes from generation to generation—such as when to harvest food based on lunar observations, how to produce heat-treated weaponry, and how to create symbolic art—likely required the use of language.

Language is not a uniquely human endeavor. Birds, dolphins, insects, monkeys, and all kinds of creatures use their own unique languages to communicate. But human language emerged to a complexity that enabled homo sapiens to quickly jump to the top of the food chain and create civilizations, art, and technologies unlike anything that came before.

Linguists traditionally believed that human language gradually evolved from caveman grunts to the type of mumbling and pointing that goes on at the dentist's office and then eventually to the complex discussions we are capable of having today. But in recent studies, some linguists are challenging that gradualistic view.[78] Instead, they believe human language arose very rapidly around 100,000 years ago from the integration of two pre-adapted systems—one from birdsongs and the other from the calls of non-human primates. Instead of a long, slow process when individual words were created and then we strung them together until sentences and paragraphs were born, Shigeru Miyazawa, a professor of linguistics at the Massachusetts Institute of Technology, explains that single words reveal traces of syntax showing they must be descended from an older, syntax-laden system. If Miyazawa is correct, then human language was created in one quick brush stroke of evolution.

Our search for milligram doses of iodine in the homo sapien

---

[78] Nobrega, Vitor A.; Miyazawa, Shigeru. "The precedence of syntax in the rapid emergence of human language in evolution as defined by the integration hypothesis," *Frontiers in Psychology*, Mar 18, 2015.

diet ends here at the birthplace of human language roughly 100,000 years ago when our ancestors moved to the sea and began building the modern human civilization we are part of today. This convergence of events in the sapien story is not coincidental. Iodine has an undeniable affect on human cognition. The World Health Organization ranks a lack of dietary iodine as the single greatest cause of intellectual disability.[79] Meanwhile, the Iodine Doctors report cases of their patients on iodine supplementation giving birth to children with IQ scores thirty points higher than either of their parents.[80]

The Fluoride Action Network identified 56 studies that investigate the relationship between fluoride and human intelligence.[81] Of those 56 studies, none of which were carried out in the United States, 49 found that fluoride exposure is associated with reduced intelligence, especially when combined with an iodine-deficient diet.[82] When researchers from Harvard conducted a meta-analysis of the literature, they concluded that the evidence was too great to ignore and that fluoride's neurotoxic effect on the human brain should be a "high research priority."[83]

Iodine should also be considered in those studies. When homo sapiens were forced to live off the sea for tens of thousands of years, it set into motion a cascade of creativity that currently manifests as space stations, supercomputers, symphonies, and nation states. I, too, experienced the rush of creative linguistic energy that comes with

---

[79] de Benoist, Bruno et. al. "Iodine deficiency in 2007: Global progress since 2003," *Food and Nutrition Bulletin*, vol 29, issue 3, 2008.

[80] Flechas, Jorge. "Total Body Iodine Sufficiency," lecture provided at a conference of the Association for the Advancement of Restorative Medicine, Portland, OR, 2011 (available at ProjectFree.Me/Flechas).

[81] For a complete listing of the studies and their findings, see www.fluoridealert.org/studies/brain01/.

[82] For a listing of relevant studies and their findings, see www.fluoridealert. org/studies/thyroid01/.

[83] Choi, Anna L.; Sun, Guifan; Zhang, Ying; Grandjean, Philippe. "Developmental Fluoride Neurotoxicity: A Systematic Review and Meta-Analysis," *Environmental Health Perspectives*, vol. 120, issue 10, Oct 2012, pp. 1362–1368.

iodine. All at once, I had to write this book. I had to tell you my thoughts and ideas. I had to develop my voice and then use it.[84]

Other species of hominids who didn't spend millennia at the sea never evolved in this way. Neanderthals lived their 200,000-year existence in small bands of nuclear families. They did not create the complex tools, advanced symbolic art, trade networks, and intricate social structures that are characteristic of homo sapiens. In 1998, an American geographer named Jerome Dobson published a study explaining that Neanderthal sites in Europe are often located in known iodine-deficient regions and that their skeletal systems and other traits have more in common with modern-day cretins than modern-day humans.[85] He points to their thickened bones and muscles, protruding brows, and high incidence of degenerative joint disease as evidence, as well as the strange angular pattern of wear on their front teeth which he asserts was caused by a protruding tongue, another sign of congenital hypothyroidism.

Scientists have made similar observations regarding homo floresiensis, the "hobbit"-like human who lived on the Indonesian island of Flores as recently as 12,000 years ago.[86]

Isotopic analysis of Neanderthal bones reveals a dietary signature of a top-level carnivore similar to that of a hyena. Studies show their carnivorous diet was consistent over time and throughout different regions of Europe.[87] In contrast, analysis of early homo sapien bones from the same region indicates a more varied diet, particularly

---

[84] I also had to create this: www.ProjectFree.Me/Voice/.

[85] Dobson, Jerome E. "The Iodine Factor in Health and Evolution," *Geographical Review*, vol. 88, issue 1, Jan 1998, pp. 3–28.

[86] Oxnard, C; Obendorf, P.J.; Kefford, B.J. "Post-Cranial Skeletons of Hypothyroid Cretins Show a Similar Anatomical Mosaic as Homo floresiensis," *PLoS ONE*, vol. 5, issue 9, 2010.

[87] Richards, Michael P.; Trinkause, Erik. "Isotopic evidence for the diets of European Neanderthals and early modern humans," *Proceedings of the National Academy of Science of the United States of America*, vol. 106, issue 38, Sep 22, 2009, pp. 16034–16039.

from fish and shellfish, even amongst sapiens living inland. In the Upper Paleolithic era, around 50,000 to 10,000 years ago when homo sapiens first populated Europe, marine shells are commonly found hundreds of miles from their sources and were known to be worn as ornamentation by sapien hunter-gatherers who lived more than 300 miles inland.[88]

A paleo diet is well and good, but we really should specify which kind of paleolithic hominid we are trying to emulate when we calculate the iodine requirement for modern humans.

Homo sapiens weren't the first mammals to return to the sea. As they say, history has a habit of repeating itself. Ungulates are the grouping of mammals that includes horses, cows, pigs, giraffes, camels, deer, and rhinoceroses. In the 1970s, researchers in Pakistan discovered archaeological remains that show a progression of extinct ungulates who made their way to the ocean 55 million years ago.[89] They now exist as relatives of an ancient type of hippopotamus. We call them cetaceans: whales, porpoises, and dolphins.

Like homo sapiens, cetaceans developed sophisticated forms of language when they took to the sea. Their vocalizations are so intricate and alien to sapien ears that we have yet to decipher their secrets. Furthermore, cetaceans are known to use tools, compose music, and demonstrate creativity, self-awareness, complex play, and empathy. Also like homo sapiens, they created elaborate social networks and proliferated in their new environment, spreading into virtually every corner of the ocean where they have thrived for millions of years.

Sapiens and cetaceans evolved from different mammalian lineages, but we share a common path from sea to land and back to sea once again. Cetaceans grew flippers, blowholes and fins while homo sapiens sprouted oars, hulls and fishing lines. Frogs and other amphibious creatures also live at this crossroads, although in a

---

[88] Dobson, Jerome E. "The Iodine Factor in Health and Evolution," *Geographical Review*, vol. 88, issue 1, Jan 1998, pp. 3–28.

[89] https://en.wikipedia.org/wiki/Evolution_of_cetaceans

different way. It has long been known that iodine is the controlling factor that guides their metamorphosis from aquatic to terrestrial beings.[90]

Iodine is a guiding element for all vertebrates. Through her studies of dogs and other domesticated animals, evolutionary zoologist Susan Crockford from the University of Victoria in British Columbia argues that thyroid hormone creates the "rhythm of life" that delineates new species.[91] Other forms of life rely on iodine as well, from simple marine invertebrates like sponges and corals to sea urchins and unicellular planktonic algae. Sebastian Venturi, an iodine researcher in Italy, attempts the grand task of explaining the pivotal role of iodine in the evolution of life on earth, beginning with cyanobacteria, a type of blue-green algae that evolved 3.5 billion years ago with the advent of photosynthesis.[92] Venturi describes iodine as the "most ancient and powerful antioxidant" and the oldest defense mechanism against oxygen produced by some of the earliest living cells.

If there is credence to Venturi's theory, then the story of iodine is the story of life. It explains why iodine is especially important for females, why nature concentrates it in mother's milk, eggs, and placental blood, and why our hominid ancestors evolved from non-human primates when they increased their consumption of the lifeblood of other animals. It also explains why the traditional sapien diet, rich in milligram doses of iodine, produced the most creative creature to ever walk the shores of planet earth.

So that's how the thinking backwards exercise works.

---

[90] Galton, V.A. "The role of thyroid hormone in amphibian metamorphosis," *Trends in Endocrinology & Metabolism*, vol. 3, issue 3, Apr 1992. pp. 96-100.

[91] Crockford, Susan J. "Commentary: Thyroid hormone in Neandertal evolution: A natural or a pathological role?" *Geographical Review*; vol. 92, issue 1, Jan 2002, pp. 73-88.

[92] Venturi, Sebastian. "Evolutionary Significance of Iodine," *Current Chemical Biology*, vol. 5, issue 3, 2011.

*****

There's No Place Like Home

"When you feel life coming down on you like a heavy weight
And you feel this crazy society adding to the strain
Take a stroll to the nearest water's edge, remember your place
Many moons have risen and fallen long, long before you came
So which way is the wind blowing?
What does your heart say?"

—Xavier Rudd, *Follow the Sun*

I didn't tell you how the story ends. After the woman runs down the mountain shouting *"Arigato zaisho"* to the trees and birds and boulders as they pass, she runs straight to the cave on the outskirts of the village where the wise healer is awaiting her return. Reaching into her pack, the woman pulls out the silver hair she plucked from the black bear's chest and presents it to the healer who eyes it closely. The wise healer then takes the hair from the woman's hand and throws it into the fire where it quickly turns to ash.

"No!" the woman cries. "What about the cure for my husband?"

The wise healer looks at her calmly. "Don't worry, all is well," she says. "Do you remember how you climbed the mountain?" The woman shakes her head yes for she remembered every step. "Do you remember how you approached the bear?" Again, the woman confirms that she does.

"Good," the wise healer assures her. "Now go home and proceed the same way with your husband."

The underlying story of this book is not about iodine or fluoride or even acne. It is a story about a woman climbing a mountain. As Clarissa explains in her telling of "The Bear," "[H]ealing

252

is in the process of questing and practice, not in a single idea." The silver hair is a talisman, a way to remember what one has learned. It is a treasure one travels far to unearth. Nothing less, but nothing more.

And what did I learn on my journey to heal my acne? I learned that the magical ingredient for the cure to acne isn't found on the bear's chest, in a pill, or at the doctor's office. It is found right here in my own home. It is in the decisions I make about where to live and where to move to when the climate changes. When to climb and when to rest. What to eat, drink, and allow to cross the threshold at my front doorstep. I learned that in ages past, our ancestors developed a sophisticated form of hunger that didn't just tell them when to eat, it told them *what* to eat. They listened as their bodies revealed the secrets of the foods they chose to consume. Now those secrets are largely forgotten, but sapien society is adept at the act of remembering. And we can still listen, too.

Will I ever be acne-proof? I don't know. But as of now, it doesn't matter. The ability to detect fluoride isn't a bad superpower to possess. Will iodine prove to be the ultimate antidote for acne? Again, I don't know. There is much study that needs to be carried out before we will be able to make that determination. These aren't studies that involve statistical analysis of rat thyroids and rabbit fur. Our tools and methods are much more direct than that. A glass of water and a mirror will do. Patience and persistence are also helpful. As Clarissa says in *Women Who Run With the Wolves*, "We can have all the knowledge in the universe, and it comes down to one thing: practice. It comes down to going home and step-by-step implementing what we know. As often as necessary, and for as long as possible, or forever, whichever comes first."

The bear is the real star of our story. He represents the dual aspects of resurrection: hibernation and awakening. Like a bear rising from a long winter's nap, now that my skin and mind are both clear I am finally able to stretch my paws to the sky and inhabit this wide-awake world the way a sapien woman is meant to do. To live a healthy

253

life as nature intended—that is my wish for all the earth's creatures including you, my sapien friend. Before my encounter with the bear, I was caged by confusion. The more I tried to climb, the harder I banged my head against the bars. Now the confusion is lifted, the cage dissolved, and I can see the path clearly, both the one we took to get here and the one that leads to where we want to go.

When her quiet hibernation draws to a close, this is when a female bear gives birth to her cubs. She wakes up ready to breath new life into the world around her. I woke up like this.

AFTERWORD: ENDING ACNE

"Like a small boat on the ocean
Setting big waves into motion"

—Rachel Platten, *Fight Song*

SO THERE YOU HAVE MY STORY OF ACNE, MY ANEKDOTA. Although I guess technically it's not an anekdota anymore—an unpublished story —presuming that if these words made their way to you it is because my story has been published.

I am about to stuff these pages in a bottle and send them off to literary agents and editors and anyone who might be willing to help me deliver them to you. I must admit, the idea of sending this book out into the world scares me a little. I just wrote a lot of words, and I'm sure some of them offended someone, some of them aren't as funny as I thought they were at the time, some of them are wrong, and some of them might spark discussions I don't want to be a part of. Intelligence analysts like myself value our quiet cubes and our anonymity. But I learned not to want the quiet of the room with no one around to find me out. There's too much going on in the world for me to stay in my cube. I'm done with it.

Your story of acne is the one that really matters. If the ideas I put forward in these pages don't resonate with your experience of the world, then I just wasted four months and all my vacation days on writing a comic tragedy about raisins. Your story will decide the fate of mine. Will my ideas be crucified by the dental cult of fluoristanism? Whacked by dermatologist drug lords? Will they be the subject of a smear campaign by conniving mink oil manufacturers? And what will Dr. Oz and Matthew McConaughey think of all this?

If this book doesn't help you heal your acne in a way that makes you want to tell other people about it, then my story about fluoride and acne ends here, and I will sink back into the shadows of my cubicle walls. But if these words changed your skin for the better, if you studied the ideas and the references and the footnotes and found them plausible, then our combined stories will reveal that all of this time while we've been trying to treat our acne, we've been dancing around the lies we tell. Our experience of acne will shine a light on the myth that fluoride is safe and effective, and I can tell you that when the lights come on we'll be ready for this.

  Don't you think it's boring how people talk? This is not one of those books where I talk about something bad going on in our torn-up town and then give you obscure suggestions for little things you can do to help fix it. This is one of those books where we fix it. Together. Fast.

  In the Appendix that follows, you will see my 7-step plan to end fluoridation. Don't be deceived by its simplicity. As Leonardo da Vinci once said, simplicity is the ultimate sophistication. The first two steps of the plan will be completed by the time you read this, steps 3 to 5 are the most important (that's your part), and the last two steps will be crazy fun to do together. Notice each phase of the plan gets easier and none of them involve arguing with anyone or trying to change someone's mind.

  Ending fluoridation will not be a fight and it's certainly not a war. It's more like breaking up with someone. In the dating world, when you realize a certain partner isn't right for you, we all know it is counterproductive to try to change them into who you want them to be, especially if they aren't eager to change. In this situation, it is best to move on. You'll need a recovery period, a time to find your footing (step 1) and heal festering wounds (step 2). It is healthy to talk with your friends about what went wrong in the relationship (step 3), and if things were really bad, you might need to request a restraining order (step 4) and find a support group to help you through it (step 5). Before you know it, you will be back out on the town again living it up (step 6) and looking to find someone new (step 7).

Growing up and growing old in this cynical sapien society our ancestors left us with, it is easy to become overwhelmed with all the negative stories that surround us. It is easy to feel small and powerless and to believe that things will never change. But that would be a sad analytic error to make. Change is the one thing we can believe in. Change is constant and often unexpected. The experts continually change their minds even when they are the last to figure things out.

Fluoride *will* go the way of lead paint, asbestos, DDT, tobacco, and mercury-poisoned hatters. Someday psychologists will publish assessments in peer-reviewed journals of the twentieth century fluoride craze. Pictures of a rare skin condition called acne will be included in health history textbooks, a required class for all sapien adolescents. After all these years struggling with acne, won't it be fun to be a part of that change? We could sit back and let someone else make the change we want to see in the world, but I decided I'm doing this for the thrill of it, killing it—never not chasing a million things I want.

The Smithsonian Institute didn't recognize the Wright Flyer as the first manned airplane until 1942. That didn't change the fact that the Wright brothers first flew it forty years prior. Smithsonian officials didn't want to embarrass their dead bureaucrats and tarnish the Institute's scientific reputation, but they were eventually forced to concede when a journalist threatened to write about the controversy in the Wright brother's biography. What does this morsel of aviation history tell us? It tells us that the bureaucrats might have bigger voices than you and I do, but they are scared of us.

Promoters of fluoridation are scared too many of us will see through their story and then they will be forced to face the unthinkable: that their policies have been poisoning millions of people for generations. The current generation of dentists will likely never admit this, but that doesn't matter. Our goal isn't to convince our ex to admit he's a jerk. Our goal is to end it and move on.

We don't need to convince everyone that fluoridation must

end. Some people can't imagine questioning the current dental authorities, and most people won't care about it at all. We just need to reach the tipping point which researchers estimate is between 15 and 18 percent market penetration. Fluoride activists like the Fluoride Action Network, Joe Mercola, David Brownstein, Erin Brockovich and others are already working to reach that magic number. When we add our voices to theirs, the tipping point will tip. Then it's a switch flipped. It's a moon eclipsed. The fluoridation myth will crack and then shatter, leaving nothing but shards beneath our feet.

Learning how to talk about fluoride in an intelligent, confident way is a critical step in the plan. I used to be embarrassed to tell people about my "fluoride allergy," but experience has shown me that once they know more of the details, most people see right through the lies bureaucrats tell. In my casual conversations with friends, family members, and coworkers about fluoride, I've found that there's one little-known secret that easily conveys the rest of the story. It's the fact that the fluoride added to the public water supply is gathered directly from the smokestacks of the phosphate fertilizer industry. For those of us who aren't caught up in their love affair with fluoride, this one fact is an ominous sign that fluoridation is a bad idea.

When you tell people that the fluoride in their drinking water is a toxic industrial waste product that Erin Brockovich herself came out swinging against, they will know fluoride isn't a story about white teeth teens.[1] They will know it's a pollution story. They will know the players. They will know the game. And they will know how the story must end.

Here's why the way things change is about to change, and why we'll always win at this. We tell ourselves science is king, but our understanding of the world is shaped through story. Historians have a theory that the way society is structured is a reflection of the primary means of communication. Since the advent of sapien language, the storytellers have wielded disproportionate influence over everyone

---

[1] To read Erin Brockovich's thoughts on fluoride, see ProjectFree.Me/Erin.

else. When we abandoned oral tradition for written myths that only a few powerful people could code and decode, our communities grew and became more hierarchical and dogmatic. Then with the printing press and the rise of literacy, we saw the birth of democracy. Television and radio ushered in corporate fairytales in the guise of cartoon tigers and commercial breaks.

Looking back over recorded history, we can see the primary means of storytelling has been largely one-sided. Someone with a megaphone speaks, drowning out the rest of us. Our top-down societies are a reflection of this type of communication. The government issues a guideline about how much fluoride your town should add to the water supply or how much iodine your doctor should recommend for your diet, and we have little choice but to listen. We can reject their guidelines on an individual level, but when we try to talk back, our tiny voices are virtually incapable of being heard.

But peer-reviewed journal articles, books from elitist publishers, and expensive network television and radio airtime are no longer our society's primary means of storytelling. Nothing like Internet has ever existed. Now the dentists post their story online, then I tell a story about their story in an ebook, and then other people tell their stories about my story about the dentist's story in the review section on Amazon. People won't read my story unless your story indicates it's worth their time. That's power. Now we're in the ring.

Sharing information is only a fraction of Internet's potential. In 1977 the United States held a Congressional hearing on the science of fluoridation after reports surfaced of a greater incidence of cancer deaths in fluoridated communities. Congress ordered the U.S. Public Health Service to have an independent contractor, Battelle Laboratory, conduct animal studies to determine if fluoride is a carcinogen. The American public continued to consume fluoride while the studies were being conducted even though the final report took 13 years to produce.

When the study was finally released, the controversial findings were the reason William Marcus, a toxicologist at the EPA's Office of Drinking Water, was fired in 1992 after raising concerns that the results show fluoride causes cancer. After a two-year legal battle, a judge ordered that Marcus be reinstated under the Whistleblower Protection Act but his concerns over fluoride were never addressed.

In June 2000, Bill Hirzy, vice president of the EPA union of professional employees, testified on behalf of the union before the United States Senate to call for a moratorium on fluoridation until the evidence that fluoride causes cancer could be independently evaluated.[2] The moratorium never happened and neither did the cancer review. This will not do.

Internet was still a kid when all this happened and so was I, but we've both done a lot of growing up since then. Politicians are easily distracted. They have many pressing matters to attend to (you know, such as campaign financing, sex scandals, and pet projects for their loudest, i.e. wealthiest, constituents—some of them even have real governing to do). But my friends and I, we cracked the code. We'll never be royals, but we can be even more powerful. We can have the power to change things the way we want things to change, and Internet is the trusty sidekick who will help us do it.

On December 2, 2015, one month ago as I write this, the U.S. National Toxicology Program held a hearing on the studies that indicate fluoride is a neurotoxin. They agreed the effects of fluoride on the developing brain are a "medium-to-high priority" and made plans to move forward with further research. If the U.S. National Toxicology Program is investigating fluoride as a neurotoxin, wouldn't it be wise for the U.S. Department of Health and Human Services to stop advising local governments to add fluoride to drinking water while they try to figure it out? Seems like a reasonable request, right? Here's your chance to ask it to the people who can make it happen.

I set up a petition at Change.org to tell the U.S. government to stop recommending the addition of fluoride to public water supplies

---

[2] To view Hirzy's presentation to Congress, see ProjectFree.Me/Hirzy.

until the neurotoxic and other negative health effects of fluoride are fully studied by toxicologists, not dentists. Each time someone signs the petition, it will be delivered to the members of the Senate Subcommittee on Wildlife, Fisheries, and Drinking Water—the same committee Bill Hirzy testified in front of fifteen years ago.

Of course Dan Sullivan, the current subcommittee chairman, won't care about my petition if I'm the only one who signs it. But I've done the initial analysis and there are a lot of people who are concerned about fluoridation. It might take some time to gain momentum, but I don't mind killing time as long as it's with you. Our voices are dispersed and therefore difficult to make out, but if we focus them on one point in the Internet ether we will hear their true volume like an orchestra coming into tune. At that moment, I suspect we will realize we are bigger than we ever dreamed.

This is the start of how it all ends.

To sign the petition, please visit:

www.ProjectFree.Me/STOP

Find table space to say your social graces
Bow your head, they're pious here, but you and I, we're pioneers
We make our own rules, our own room, no bias here
Let 'em sell what they are sellin', there are no buyers here

So gather all the rebels now
We'll rebel rouse and sing aloud
We don't care what they say, no way
And we will leave the empty chairs
To those who say we can't sit there
We're fine all by ourselves

We brought our drum and this is how we dance
No mistaking, we make our breaks, if you don't like our 808s
Then leave us alone, cause we don't need your policies
We have no apologies for being

Find me where the wild things are...

We will carve our place into time and space
We will find our way, or we'll make a way
Find your great, don't you hide your *face*
Let it shine, shine, shine, shine, shine, shine

—Alessia Cara, *Wild Things*

Appendix: The Plan

Step 1. ~~Write a book to tell people about fluoride and acne~~ —Me

Step 2. ~~Create a website to help people with acne~~ —Me   *Please do this one!

www.ProjectFree.Me/Resources
(go here for the cheat sheets)

Step 3. Help spread the word about fluoride and acne —You

> ‣ review The End of Acne on Amazon
> ‣ share success stories at **acne@ProjectFree.Me**
> ‣ tweet #**TheEndofAcne** (I'm **@MelissaGardner_**)

Step 4. Tell the U.S. government to stop recommending fluoride until the negative health effects are fully studied by toxicologists —Us

www.ProjectFree.Me/STOP
(you will be redirected to the petition at Change.org)

Step 5. Join the ProjectFree email group at **www.ProjectFree.Me/Email** to make sure Congress follows through —You

Step 6. Party like pop stars when we end fluoridation! —Us

*preferably in person, location TBD
(prob. where the wild things are)

Step 7. Decide what part of this torn-up town we will fix next —Us

References

BELOW IS A LIST OF REFERENCES FOR *The End of Acne* in addition to those included in the footnotes. They are mentioned in their order of appearance in the text. For a complete list of references, including links when available, visit **ProjectFree.Me/References.**

*****

Chabris, Christopher and Daniel Simons. *The Invisible Gorilla: How Our Intuitions Deceive Us.* New York: Random House, Inc., 2009.

Kahneman, Daniel. *Thinking Fast and Slow.* New York: Farrar, Straus and Giroux, 2011.

Greene, Robert. *Mastery.* New York: The Penguin Group, 2012.

Cordain, L., *The Dietary Cure for Acne,* Fort Collins, CO: Paleo Diet Enterprises, LLC, 2006.

Berkun, Scott. *The Myths of Innovation.* Sebastapol, Canada: O'Reilly Media, 2010.

Cialdini, Robert. *Influence: The Psychology of Persuasion.* New York: Harper Business, 1984.

Connett, Paul et al. *The Case Against Fluoride.* White River Junction, VT: Chelsea Green Publishing, 2010.

Hanlon, Patrick. *Primal Branding: Create Zealots for Your Brand, Your Company, and Your Future.* New York: Free Press, 2006.

Bryson, Christopher. *The Fluoride Deception.* New York: Seven Stories Press, 2011.

Bernays, E.L. *Propaganda*. New York: Horace Liveright, 1928.

Bernays, Edward L., *Biography of an Idea: Memoirs of Public Relations Counsel*. Simon and Schuster, 1965.

Grant, Tara. *The Hidden Plague: A Field Guide For Surviving and Overcoming Hidradenitis Suppurativa*. Malibu, CA: Primal Blueprint Publishing, 2013.

Diaz, Cameron. *The Body Book*. New York: Harper Collins Publishers, 2013.

Wilson, Lawrence. *Sauna Therapy for Detoxification and Healing*. L.D. Wilson Consultants, Inc., 2011.

Farrow, Lynne. *The Iodine Crisis: What You Don't Know About Iodine Can Wreck Your Life*. Devon Press, 2013.

Brownstein, David. *Iodine: Why You Need It, Why You Can't Live Without It*. 4th ed. West Bloomfield, MI: Medical Alternatives Press, 2009.

Bryun, G.W. and Charles M. Poser. *The History of Tropical Neurology: Nutritional Disorders*. Science History Publications, 2003.

Pinkola Estes, Clarissa. *Women Who Run With the Wolves: Myths and Stories of the Wild Woman Archetype*. New York: Random House Publishing Group, 1992.

Price, Weston A. *Nutrition and Physical Degeneration*. New York: Harper & Brothers, 1939.

ACKNOWLEDGEMENTS

SINCE THIS IS A SELF-PUBLISHED BOOK, I don't have the normal laundry list of publishing people to thank for helping me bring it into the world. There was no agent. No team of professionals at a publishing house. Not even a cover designer. But of course, I literally have *millions* of people to thank. These are just a few of them.

Thank you to the good people at Google who lay a universe of information at the feet of my curious mind. Wikipedia, same. Thank you to the Fluoride Action Network for posting insane amounts of information about fluoride online. I never could have figured out how to heal my acne without it. Thank you to the Iodine Doctors and others like them who put their reputations and careers on the line every day for their patients by questioning the established health dogma. Thank you to Amazon for connecting me with the books and products I needed to put my theories to the test, and then for creating a home for my book when the time came to write about it all. Thank you to Apple for giving me the tools I needed to gather all that information and assemble it into a finished product. I will love you forever or until something better comes along. You know how it goes.

To my writing coach, Stephen Harrod Buhner, thanks for teaching me how to follow a golden thread.[1] I yanked that thread until the whole story unravelled and then I used it to sew a sparkly gold dress. I hope you like it. To Keith Blount for creating Scrivener and Tim Ferris for taking the time to tell me about it. Sitting down to write your first book is daunting, but that dang Scrivener tutorial... thank you.

Thank you to Hardy Limeback for all your encouragement and support. Someday I will tell the story of the first time you emailed me and people won't believe it. Thanks to Bill Hirzy and several of my analyst colleagues (you know who you are) for reading my entire

---

[1] Buhner, Stephen Harrod. *Ensouling Language: On the Art of Nonfiction and the Writer's Life.* Rochester, VT: Inner Traditions, 2010.

8,500-word exposé on raisins and providing constructive criticism. To my original blogging buddy and eventual beta reader, Elizabeth Walling of The Nourished Life, thank you for reading an early copy of the manuscript for *The End of Acne* and providing valuable feedback. You are the kind of sapien woman who reminds me to be proud to be a sapien woman.

To my editor, Darlene Musso, thank you for conspiring with me on this project, for sharing your candid thoughts and ideas, for loving me like I grew up as part of the family, and for the perfect Christmas card you sent before you even knew I was writing a book about Inuits and cetaceans and language and the ocean.[2] It hung above my writing desk and inspired me every day. In case anyone was in doubt, this is hard proof you are an angel.

Thank you to my parents for telling me when I was a little girl (before I was old enough to mistake truth for cliché) that I can do anything I set my mind to. Thanks for the happiness in your voice when I call you on the phone and you realize it's me on the other side of the line. For how excited I know you will be when I tell you I wrote a book. For thinking the world of me. For your endless love. For all that and more. Thank you. It worked.

To sweet Gia, who reminds me every day that homo sapiens are not the only beings being. And to my Marco who passed by me for ten years before finally saying hello. I'm so glad you said hello. That was the moment everything changed. Thank you for feeding me while I wrote this book. And for listening to me talk about raisins. And for never getting tired (or at least pretending not to get tired) of listening to me talk about raisins. I always say you are my dream man. But in truth, I could not have dreamed of a man as perfect for me as you are.

Finally, to everyone past and future who reads my story and realizes it's their own. Your testimonials are the reason this book exists. They are the reason I do this work. Thank you for sharing them with me. Thank you for reading even to this very last word. :)

---

[2] www.ProjectFree.Me/Writing-Inspiration

THE BEGINNING

OF

THE END

But please, let's not make this goodbye.

www.ProjectFree.Me/Email

CPSIA information can be obtained
at www.ICGtesting.com
Printed in the USA
LVOW13s1835170817
545388LV00013B/1209/P